The Green Smoothie Recipe Book

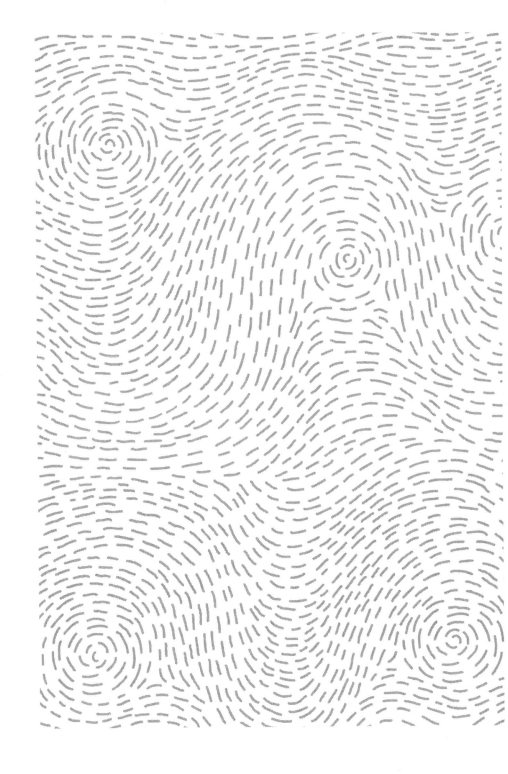

THE
GREEN
SMOOTHIE
RECIPE BOOK

over

100

HEALTHY GREEN SMOOTHIE RECIPES
to LOOK *and* FEEL AMAZING

MENDOCINO PRESS

Contents

Green Smoothie Recipes

Chapter Five: Green Smoothies for Beginners

Chapter Six: Breakfast Smoothies

Chapter Seven: Super Green (Fruit-Free) Smoothies

Chapter Eight: Smoothies for Weight Loss

Chapter Nine: Detox and Cleansing Smoothies

Chapter Ten: Smoothies for Digestive Health

Chapter Eleven: Smoothies for Healthy Skin and Hair

Chapter Twelve: Green Energy

Chapter Thirteen: Low-Fat Smoothies

Chapter Fourteen: Green Smoothies Kids Will Love

Appendix: Know Your Produce

References   181

Index   183

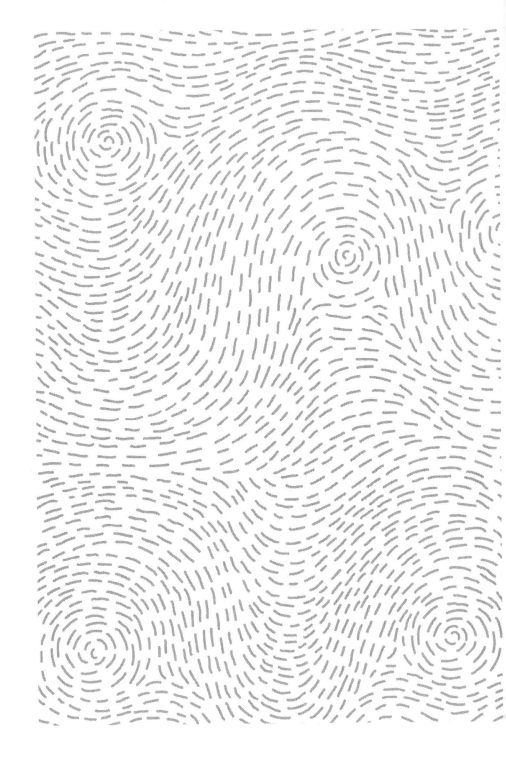

Introduction

Your overall well-being depends greatly on what you eat, and of all foods, fruits and vegetables are among the healthiest. Eating enough of them every day can be a challenge, though. That's where green smoothies come in. Quick and easy to make with just a few simple tools, these smoothies contain several servings of fruits and vegetables apiece, making it much easier to ensure you are getting the nutrition you need.

The Green Smoothie Recipe Book contains all the information you need to start making green smoothies, from which tools you will need, to tips for making the process quick and convenient, to easy methods for preparing and storing a wide variety of fruits and vegetables. You will also discover easy methods for adding superfoods to the smoothies you make, plus you'll find plenty of ideas for making recipes more exciting with simple spices.

In this book, you'll also find practical information on the importance of fruits and vegetables in the daily diet. You will learn why it is important to eat a wide variety of plant-based foods, and you will discover how consuming them can benefit your overall health and even improve your appearance.

With over a hundred recipes to follow, including smoothies for beginners, low-fat and low-sugar options, and even nutritious, kid-friendly smoothies that will please the pickiest palates, this informative guide is fun and easy to use.

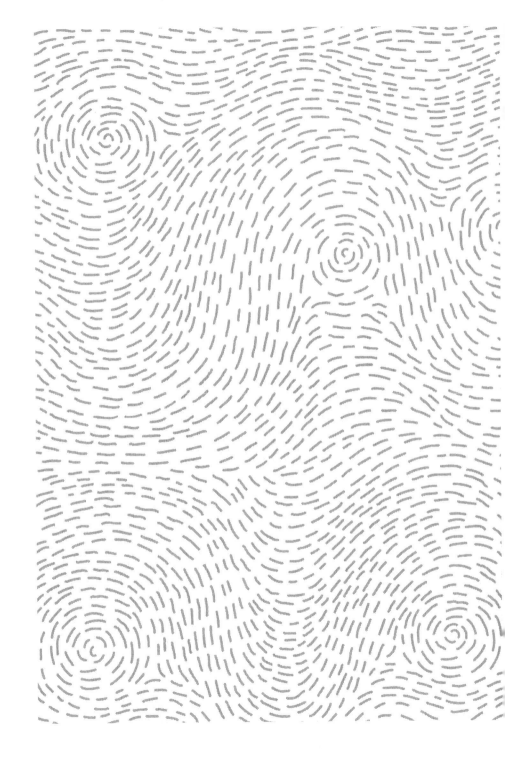

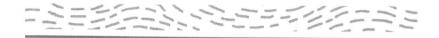

PART ONE

Green Smoothie Mania

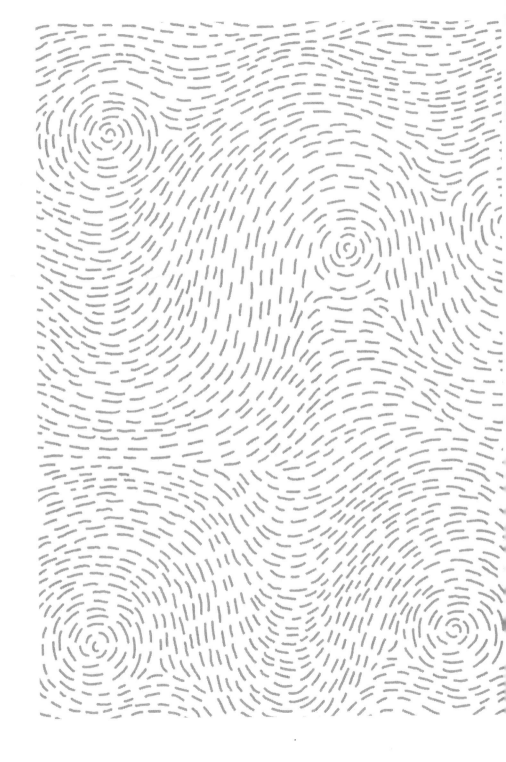

CHAPTER ONE

Green Smoothie Basics

It's not at all surprising that green smoothies have become so popular. Busy lifestyles demand quick, filling foods that are easy to consume on the go. But most fast-food contributes to obesity, high blood pressure, and other health woes. Current dietary guidelines published by the U.S. government emphasize three major nutritional goals for everyone:

1. Balance calorie intake and physical activity to better manage weight.
2. Increase consumption of whole, healthy foods, especially fruits and vegetables.
3. Consume fewer processed foods, such as those that contain refined grains, added sugars, cholesterol, trans fats, saturated fats, and sodium.

Not surprisingly, adding green smoothies to your daily diet can help you to meet these goals while making sure you don't go hungry. Sometimes it's not practical to eat a bowl of fruits and vegetables, but replacing unhealthy snacks and fast-food meals with green smoothies is an easy way to ensure that you are getting at least the minimum—if not more—of the natural foods that are best for your body.

WHAT ARE GREEN SMOOTHIES?

Green smoothies are usually blended combinations of various fruits and vegetables, although some low-sugar recipes contain no fruit at all. All green smoothies contain leafy green vegetables, such as kale or spinach, though it's often impossible to taste the greens beneath the flavors of the fruits, nut butters, and other delicious—and healthy—ingredients that can be added.

Any vegetable or fruit can be incorporated into a green smoothie recipe; whether you enjoy tropical tastes from such fruits as pineapples and papayas or you prefer savory flavors such as spicy jalapeños, ripe tomatoes, and bell peppers, you'll find plenty of opportunities to satisfy your cravings with healthy, homemade smoothies.

Unlike some commercially available drinks that are green in color, green smoothies have no artificial colors. And as long as you use all natural ingredients, they have no artificial flavors, either. Herbs such as mint, cilantro, parsley, and basil intensify the smoothies' flavors and colors, and almond or coconut milk, yogurt, or even green tea can be added to enhance both taste and nutritional value.

SMOOTHIES VERSUS JUICE

While fresh juices are made with many of the same ingredients, smoothies contain more dietary fiber. Plus, they can be made with foods that are difficult to incorporate into juices, including avocados, bananas, nuts, and more.

Because fruit juices contain less fiber, they are typically much higher on the glycemic index than smoothies are. The glycemic index is a ranking of carbohydrates according to how much they raise your blood sugar levels after you've eaten them. Foods with a high glycemic index are absorbed more rapidly by the body, but also lead to a "crash" when their energy is quickly used up. Foods with a low glycemic index, such as green smoothies, provide a steadier, longer-lasting energy supply. In addition, the fiber in smoothies helps promote a feeling of fullness that juices don't provide. While fresh homemade juices do offer excellent nutrition, they are not normally as satisfying as green smoothies.

Finally, green smoothies are considered to be complete foods due to their fiber content, while juices are incomplete foods.

Fresh juices are excellent to add to smoothies. If you enjoy juicing now, you don't have to give up your habit. Instead, make a little extra juice to use in place of some or all of the water or other liquid in smoothie recipes. Citrus juice, berry juice, mixed fruit juice, and even green juice made without fruit can greatly enhance your smoothies' flavors and nutritional value.

THE SCIENCE BEHIND GREEN SMOOTHIES

Most of the nutritional value of fruits and vegetables is held within the plants' cell walls. These structures are often quite tough, and most of us do not chew our food well enough to access all the nutrition that's warehoused inside the plants we eat. While the digestive process does break down some of the fiber, giving us access to these nutrients, many are swept right through our bodies.

When you blend fruits and vegetables, more cell walls are destroyed, unlocking more nutrition, including the amino acids that are necessary for increased protein production and improved metabolism.

Nutritionists have been urging people to eat more fruits, leafy greens, and other vegetables for decades, particularly because the standard American diet is sorely lacking in the nutrients that raw plants contain. While it is true that a healthy diet high in fresh, raw foods isn't a solution for all ailments, it does improve the immune system and contribute to overall well-being, particularly when undesirable foods are eliminated.

GREEN SMOOTHIES FOR HEALTH

Green smoothies have many other health benefits. The more often you enjoy green smoothies, the more of these benefits you will reap.

Safe, Natural Weight Loss

By replacing high-calorie foods that are relatively devoid of nutrients with green smoothies, you can lose weight quickly and easily. While low-calorie diets are often woefully low in nutrition, green smoothies contain more than enough of the vitamins and minerals your body needs to function at its best, ensuring that your dieting will do no harm.

Since replacing unhealthy snacks and fast-food meals with green smoothies can often lead to rapid weight loss, be sure to do some weight-bearing exercise each day to improve muscle tone. This will help to reduce the appearance of sagging skin while you lose weight. Focus on strengthening your arms, legs, and core for best results.

Reduced Sugar Absorption

Consuming too much sugar is at least partially to blame for many health problems, including diabetes, obesity, and heart disease. The high concentration of fiber in green vegetables and fruits aids in slowing and regulating the absorption of sugar from the foods we eat.

Increased Fruit and Vegetable Intake

The American Cancer Society recommends we eat between five and nine servings of vegetables and fruits daily to help prevent cancer and other common diseases. Green smoothies make it easy to get the recommended amount of fruits and vegetables.

Improved Antioxidant and Phytonutrient Intake

Antioxidants are primarily found in plants, and phytonutrients are found naturally only in plants. Together, these nutritional compounds may protect your cells against the effects of free radicals. Free radicals are molecules that can damage cells and may play a role in heart disease, cancer, and other diseases. The compounds also may help boost your immune system and improve your resistance to illness.

Increased Chlorophyll Intake

Chlorophyll is the green pigment found in all plants. This pigment drives photosynthesis—a plant's process of using the energy from the sun to transform water and carbon dioxide into oxygen and carbohydrates. When we eat foods containing high levels of chlorophyll, we improve tissue oxygenation within our bodies, improving our immune response.

Increased Energy

When you focus on eating whole, natural foods, your energy levels increase markedly, thanks to the combination of vitamins, minerals, and other nutrients these foods contain. Since fruits and vegetables don't bog down your digestive system, you feel lighter and more energetic when you eat them regularly.

Improved Focus and Greater Mental Clarity

When you improve your diet, you also gain a greater ability to focus, and you improve your mental clarity. If you decide to eliminate excess caffeine from your routine, as many who enjoy green smoothies regularly do, you will also reduce stress and anxiety levels.

Better Sleep

Vegetables and fruits are natural sources of tryptophan, which is a substance that aids in relaxation. If you rely on over-the-counter or prescription medications for sound sleep now, you may discover you can eliminate them from your routine after embracing the green smoothie habit.

Reduced Sugar and Carbohydrate Cravings

Cravings for unhealthy foods can be very difficult to overcome. The body craves the nutrients it is lacking, and we tend to misinterpret these cravings as a strong desire for things such as chocolate, pizza, or macaroni and cheese. When you nourish your body with green smoothies, you reduce these cravings. After drinking green smoothies for a few weeks, you will find that you crave healthier foods instead of junk.

Alkalizing the Body

Many processed foods, meats, and products that contain high levels of animal protein can produce acid, which raises the pH level of the blood, in turn causing the body to leach calcium from the bones. Vegetables and fruits do the opposite, alkalizing the body (lowering the pH) and possibly decreasing your risk of developing osteoporosis.

Improved Sexual Function

One unexpected way fruits and vegetables can enhance your health is by improving sexual function. Folate, carotenoids, fiber, magnesium, and other plant nutrients are necessary for a healthy reproductive system. In addition, hypertension can contribute to sexual dysfunction. Reducing the potential for this problem by enjoying green smoothies is an easy, drug-free way to keep libido strong.

TOP TEN BENEFITS OF GREEN SMOOTHIES

Green smoothies provide numerous benefits, and the more often you drink them, the greater your chances of enjoying these benefits. Here are just a few of the beneficial ways green smoothies can work for you. If you drink them often, you may find that the green smoothie:

1. **Slows the aging process.** Taking in plenty of antioxidants is a good way to slow damage that occurs over time. While there is no way to stop aging altogether, a green smoothie habit can help slow it from the inside out.
2. **Improves digestion.** Fruits and vegetables contain fiber, pectin, and other macronutrients that contribute to healthy digestion. Problems ranging from acid indigestion to irregularity are likely to decrease or disappear when you drink green smoothies regularly.
3. **Reduces mood swings.** The nutrients in the foods we eat can affect our emotions. Tryptophan, magnesium, folate, and other B vitamins that are abundant in leafy greens can help keep you on an even keel. This is partly because eating fruits and vegetables throughout the day helps keep the body fueled while maintaining stable blood sugar levels.
4. **Eliminates toxins.** Toxins are all around us. They are in the foods we eat, the water we drink, and the air we breathe. Depending on your diet and environment, your toxic load could be quite high. The fruits

and vegetables in green smoothies help maximize the body's efficiency, making it easier to flush toxins from the body.

5. **Optimizes hydration.** Many people are chronically dehydrated. While it's important to drink plenty of water each day, increasing the amount of food that contains pure water is also important for proper hydration. Fruits and vegetables are made up mostly of water, and they also contain the electrolytes our bodies need to regulate all sorts of functions.

6. **Improves skin tone.** When we're tired, dehydrated, and stressed, our skin suffers. Eating unhealthy processed foods that increase toxin loads takes a toll on skin, too. When your body is able to eliminate toxins, and when you are properly nourished, your skin will show it. By drinking green smoothies regularly, you can improve your appearance from the inside out.

7. **Satisfies hunger with minimal calories.** Basic green smoothies are very low in calories, yet they satisfy hunger while providing you with a long-lasting source of energy. Adding a bit of protein to your smoothies makes them even more satisfying.

8. **Makes healthy nutrition almost effortless.** Cooking healthy food at home can be time-consuming, and purchasing premade foods can be hard on your budget. Green smoothies are fast and easy to make, and when you use preparation shortcuts such as chopping ingredients and freezing them in advance, you can whip up a wonderful, nutritious smoothie in only a few minutes. Cleanup is easy, too.

9. **Increases the appeal of vegetables.** Many children and plenty of adults dislike vegetables. If you tend to avoid vegetables and want to change that, or if you want to increase a child's vegetable intake, delicious green smoothies that taste like frozen treats are the perfect way to disguise the vegetables.

10. **Offers portability, for good nutrition anywhere.** While it is best to drink the smoothies you make immediately, it's easy to make a large batch to drink as needed. Green smoothies can be refrigerated in airtight containers for up to three days, and they are perfect for pouring into travel cups you can take along with you to work, to school, or on long drives. Having ready access to a healthy, portable meal can help you to avoid fast-foods and other unhealthy choices.

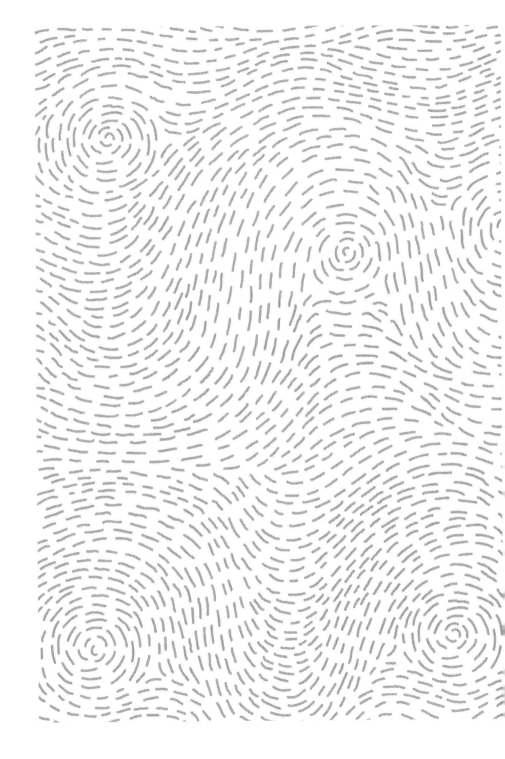

CHAPTER TWO

Going Green

Green smoothies are very easy to make, whether or not you are someone who enjoys cooking. While it is simple to make a quick, basic smoothie by throwing a few handfuls of kale or spinach into a blender, adding a peeled banana, and thinning it with a little water, using the right tools and knowing how to prepare a wide variety of fruits and vegetables to add to your smoothies can make the process much easier, giving you more incentive to try new flavors.

ESSENTIAL TOOLS FOR GETTING STARTED

You may already have the tools required for adding smoothies to your daily diet. If you don't, they are easy to find at stores that carry kitchen goods.

Blender

Blenders range widely in price. You'll find a few basic models available for around twenty dollars, but while you're researching, you'll see advertisements for blenders that cost several hundred dollars. Although budget is always a consideration, it is a good idea to look for a blender that will stand up to the rigors of regular use. If you can't afford a high-end blender right away, you can extend your blender's life by minimizing the amount of hard or frozen items you process with it.

Cutting Board

Use a different cutting board for preparing fresh produce than the one you use for cutting meat, fish, and cheese. Because green smoothies are consumed raw, it is vital that you prevent the potential for exposure to salmonella and other pathogens associated with meats and other foods that must be cooked.

Be sure to thoroughly sanitize your cutting board after each use. Wash it with an antibacterial dish soap and lots of hot water.

Sharp Knives

Sharp knives in an assortment of shapes and sizes are essential for preparing vegetables and fruits for smoothies. Have a simple knife sharpener in your drawer to keep them well honed. Basic knives to use include the following:

- **Chef's knife:** Also known as a French knife, a chef's knife has a sharp tip; a sharp, curved cutting edge; and a heavy heel that makes penetrating foods such as melons and pineapples easy. (The heel is the widest part of the knife, where the blade meets the handle.)
- **Utility knife:** Smaller and much lighter than a chef's knife, a utility knife is perfect for cutting into medium-size fruits such as mangoes, which are typically too large for a paring knife to handle.
- **Paring knife:** Paring knives are ideal for cutting heavy peels away from fruits and vegetables. They are also useful for cutting produce into small, easily managed pieces.
- **Serrated slicer:** Soft or slippery fruits and vegetables, such as persimmons, tomatoes, and peppers, are often easiest to slice with a serrated blade.

Additional Tools

While not absolutely necessary, there are some additional tools that can make preparing fresh produce easier. These include:

- A vegetable peeler for peeling a wide variety of fruits and vegetables, from carrots and cucumbers to mangoes and papayas
- A melon baller for scooping chunks of melon and other fleshy items from their skins efficiently

- A corer for quickly and efficiently removing cores from fruits such as apples and pears
- Measuring cups and measuring spoons
- Kitchen shears for quickly chopping herbs
- A colander or strainer for rinsing and draining fruits and vegetables
- A slim spatula for scraping the blender's reservoir clean
- Ice cube trays and baking sheets for easily freezing prepared smoothie ingredients

Be sure to maintain your tools. Clean and dry them after each use, taking particular care to follow the manufacturer's instructions for disassembling and washing your blender. Sharpen your knives periodically to ensure they cut through even tough-skinned fruits and vegetables with ease, and store them and other sharp-edged tools carefully to prevent nicks and other damage.

BUYING, STORING, CLEANING, AND FREEZING

While some people are familiar with a wide variety of fresh produce and are comfortable handling it, the majority of us are familiar with only a few of the most common items. Buying, storing, freezing, and cleaning produce may sound like a lot of work. Luckily, these tasks are not terribly daunting once you know what to do. Like many other things in life, the more frequently you do them, the easier they will become for you.

Buying Produce

Before setting out on your first smoothie shopping trip, take some time to review recipes and decide which ones you'd like to try. Create a shopping list, so you don't end up buying more than you need or will be able to use within a reasonable amount of time.

Depending on where you live, you may have several options for buying the ingredients you need. Local organic produce from a farmers market or co-op is great; organic items that are not grown locally are also good choices.

Conventionally grown produce often costs less than organic, but you will need to work harder to prepare it for your smoothies.

When shopping, look at dates, if applicable, and choose the items that are freshest. In addition, look for the following:

- Unblemished skin, without obvious dents, scabs, or mold
- Unbruised fruit (bruised items will need to be prepared immediately)
- Bright colors
- Firm flesh, but with a little give when squeezed
- An appropriate aroma, without any underlying sourness
- Crisp, plump leaves without large brown or wilted areas

The availability of fresh produce varies from one place to the next, so if fresh items are not available, check to see if you can buy what you want frozen. Frozen fruits and vegetables without additives contain as much nutrition as fresh ones do. In fact, they are sometimes nutritionally superior, particularly when foods are out of season or must be shipped long distances.

Storing Fresh Fruits and Vegetables

To ensure fresh fruits and vegetables keep nutrients and flavors—and stay fresh—store your produce properly. In addition, proper storage can help finish the ripening process and improve taste in certain types of produce.

- Apples, bananas, and citrus fruits can be stored on a countertop in a well-ventilated fruit bowl for three to five days, depending on ripeness.
- Make peaches, pears, apricots, and other fruits last longer by storing them in the crisper section of the refrigerator.
- Purchase melons just before using them. If you can't use them right away, it is best to refrigerate them to prevent spoilage.
- Store ripe pineapple in the refrigerator. If a pineapple isn't quite ripe, you can set it on a ventilated trivet or a baking rack on the counter at room temperature for up to a week. When the sides of the pineapple take on a yellow or tan color, the fruit is ripe and ready to be used or refrigerated.

- Cucumbers, zucchini, bell peppers, and other vegetables should be stored in the crisper section of the refrigerator. Keep a close eye on your produce and try to use it within three days of purchase. Some items might last longer, but nutrients are lost as the foods age.
- Tomatoes retain their flavor better if left unrefrigerated. Plan to use them within two or three days.
- Berries should be purchased when ripe and used right away. If you can't use all the berries you buy within two or three days, consider freezing them to prevent waste.
- Leafy greens should be stored in the crisper section of your refrigerator. Placing a folded paper towel in the bag with your greens will help them last longer by absorbing moisture. Most greens should be used within three to five days from the date of purchase.

Cleaning Produce

While you may be tempted to clean produce immediately after bringing it home, doing so can cause your food to spoil sooner. Brush off any visible dirt before storing your fruits and vegetables, but follow the rest of these steps when you are preparing your produce for smoothies or for long-term storage in the freezer.

Many vegetables and fruits are covered with layers of shellac or wax that protect them during shipping and help to prevent early spoilage. In addition, these items have often been handled several times, so the presence of contaminants, including serious viruses, is a real risk. And unless you are using organic produce, your fruits and vegetables are likely to be contaminated with pesticides and herbicides. Luckily, it is very easy to remove residue, germs, and other contaminants from produce.

Begin by thoroughly rinsing the food in clean, cool water. Scrub away visible dirt with a vegetable brush. If you're using organic produce with no wax, it will now be clean and ready to use.

If you are using conventional produce or any produce with a wax coating, the next step is to cleanse it thoroughly with a fruit and vegetable wash designed to eliminate harmful residues. You can either purchase a commercial wash or save money by making your own using the simple recipe that follows.

Fruit and Vegetable Wash

- 1 cup water
- 1 tablespoon vinegar
- 2 tablespoons baking soda

Pour all ingredients into a new spray bottle, using caution because the baking soda and vinegar will foam up when they come into contact. Cap tightly after the fizzing stops. To use, spray on fruits and vegetables. Allow the mixture to remain on the produce for five minutes, then use a vegetable brush to thoroughly remove residue. Rinse treated items under cool, running water before use.

Once your produce has been washed, it's time to cut away stems, bruised areas, and blemishes before further processing. Removing all impurities ensures you will enjoy the best flavors possible.

Many leafy greens and herbs are grown in sandy soil that leaves behind grit that can be hard to see. Unfortunately, tiny particles in the bottom of your glass completely ruin the enjoyment you get from drinking green smoothies. So submerge the greens or whole herbs in a large bowl of clean, cool water after treating them with fruit and vegetable wash. Allow them to sit for about a minute, then reach in and swish them around with your hand. Lift the vegetables out of the bowl, then pour out the water and any residue. Rinse the bowl thoroughly and repeat the process. Blot the greens or herbs dry or place them in a centrifugal salad spinner to remove the water clinging to the leaves.

Freezing Extras

There are a few reasons you may wish to freeze some of the fruits and vegetables you buy. If a certain item is on sale, you may want to buy more than you can use at once. Perhaps you enjoy icy cold smoothies and love the idea of having them each day, or maybe you need a way to save time.

Before you start, make sure you have plenty of space in your freezer for a baking sheet or two. Next, clean the items you want to freeze and cut them into chunks no larger than one inch square. The smaller the chunks are, the easier it will be for your blender to handle them.

Arrange the cut-up pieces on the baking sheet so they are not touching one another. Place the baking sheet in the freezer overnight. In the morning, transfer the frozen produce into a freezer bag. Be sure to mark the bag with the date and contents, then store it in the freezer for up to six months.

If you like, you can chop all the items needed for various smoothie recipes and freeze them as just described. Store all the ingredients for one smoothie in a single freezer bag. You can also make several smoothies at once, then pour your smoothies into ice cube trays. When the cubes have hardened, store them in freezer bags for later use. These methods enable you to make quick, easy smoothies when you are pressed for time.

When you are ready to use the items you have frozen, you can either pop them right into the blender or let them thaw slightly before blending.

TIPS FOR BETTER SMOOTHIES

Making smoothies should be fun, fast, and easy. After all, one big reason people enjoy them so much is that they are simple to prepare. But they should also be delicious. Use the following tips to enhance the taste and texture of your smoothies.

Add Ice

When the weather turns hot, a cold drink is an excellent way to cool down. Add some crushed ice to your smoothies after you have completely blended all other ingredients. As a bonus, this will help hydrate you.

Avoid Curdling

Certain acidic fruits and vegetables will cause dairy products and soy milk to curdle. One of the worst combinations is citrus fruit and soy milk. If you want a creamy, citrus-flavored green smoothie, use coconut milk or another nut milk as the liquid base.

Don't Use Plain Tap Water

Invest in a filter for your faucet or a water-filtering pitcher to keep in your refrigerator. Plain tap water sometimes tastes of chemicals, and it often contains excess chlorine and other contaminants. If you use bottled water, be sure the plastic bottles contain no BPA.

Fizz It Up

Kombucha is a lightly fizzy fermented drink made from sweetened black tea. It's delicious and healthy, and it makes an excellent addition to green smoothies. If you're craving soda or seltzer, try thinning your smoothie fifty-fifty with kombucha. Plain club soda will also add some fizz. Stir in your fizzy liquid after you've blended all the other ingredients, because a whirl in the blender will dissipate all the bubbles.

Experiment with Ingredients

Once you've learned how to make basic green smoothies, experiment with different ingredients, and try using old favorite ingredients in surprising new ways. For example, frozen coconut water makes an interesting replacement for ice cubes, plus it gives you a boost of magnesium, potassium, and electrolytes.

TEN COMMONLY ASKED QUESTIONS

1. Is it ever okay to add sweetener or sugar to a green smoothie?

Adding sugar to a green smoothie is generally not a good idea, because you're basically undoing the good of all that fresh produce. However, you can add a little local honey to your smoothie to make it sweeter, while also providing some natural allergy relief. While you should avoid artificial sweeteners, you can add some organic stevia to your smoothie to increase sweetness without adding calories or chemicals.

2. Can I lose weight or detoxify my body by going on a green smoothie fast?

Green smoothie fasts are popular, but they can be challenging. In addition, cutting calories too much can meddle with your metabolism. And you really need to know what you're doing to create a complete and balanced diet from nothing but smoothies. If you want to lose weight, replacing unhealthy foods with green smoothies should be adequate. If you are considering a green smoothie fast for detoxification purposes, consult your doctor to make sure doing so will not place your health at risk.

3. I need to gain weight, but I don't want to take traditional weight gainers. Can I use green smoothies for weight gain?

You can use green smoothies to gain weight. The best way to do this is to choose recipes that use ingredients that contain healthy fat and/or are relatively high in calories. Adding avocado, nut butters, organic coconut oil, flax oil, extra bananas, and other nutrient-dense foods to your smoothies increases their caloric value while ensuring you take in no empty calories. You can also add protein powder to smoothies for an extra boost.

4. I drank green smoothies, and now I am suffering from gas and bloating. Is this normal?

When you add plenty of green smoothies to a previously low-fiber diet, it is normal to suffer from a bit of embarrassing gas and uncomfortable bloating at first. When the gastrointestinal system encounters more fiber than usual, there can be some difficulty with digestion as excess plant matter begins to ferment in the digestive tract. This can also happen if you mix too much fat into your smoothie. To avoid gas and bloating, introduce smoothies into your diet gradually.

5. Do I absolutely *have* to put all those greens in my smoothie?

The healthy benefits of smoothies are greatly amplified by the presence of greens. They contain iron, calcium, magnesium, and several essential vitamins, including vitamin K and vitamin A. Most people eat less of these leafy greens than they should, and blending them into smoothies is the best way to sneak them into your diet. If you are having a hard time with greens, start by using just a few leaves of baby spinach in each smoothie. You will not even taste it. Keep adding the greens and trying new ones until the concept seems less alien to you.

6. How many green smoothies should I be drinking each day?

When you're first starting out, try for one sixteen-ounce green smoothie each day. Gradually increase your intake until you are drinking between two and four green smoothies daily.

7. Why does my green smoothie sometimes turn brown if I don't drink it right away?

When leafy greens and other fruits and vegetables are processed in a blender, they begin to oxidize as air molecules interact with enzymes contained within their cellular structures. This process is harmless, but it does result in colors that are less appealing to the eye. If you want to save smoothies for later and keep them bright green, you can slow natural oxidization by freezing rather than refrigerating them.

8. I want to try a recipe that calls for a fruit or vegetable that is not available where I am. Can I make substitutions?

It is fine to substitute ingredients in smoothie recipes, as long as you make sure to rotate leafy greens as recommended in Chapter Three.

9. I don't like the taste of a watered-down smoothie—it seems bland. Do I have to add water to my smoothies?

There is no need to add water to your smoothies, as long as you use some kind of liquid to prevent the blender blade from getting stuck. You can use fresh fruit juice; green or herbal tea; coconut water; soy, almond, or coconut milk; or any other liquid that is compatible with the recipe you are using. Be sure to stay away from things that contain a lot of added sugar, fat, or chemicals.

10. How long should it take me to blend a smoothie?

It depends on your blender. If you are using a high-speed blender, it may take only thirty to forty seconds to blend your smoothies. If you are using an inexpensive model that has less power, you may spend longer than ninety seconds blending your smoothies. Focus on blending until you are satisfied with the end results. The more often you make smoothies, the more familiar you will become with the process and the easier it will be to determine when your drink is ready to enjoy.

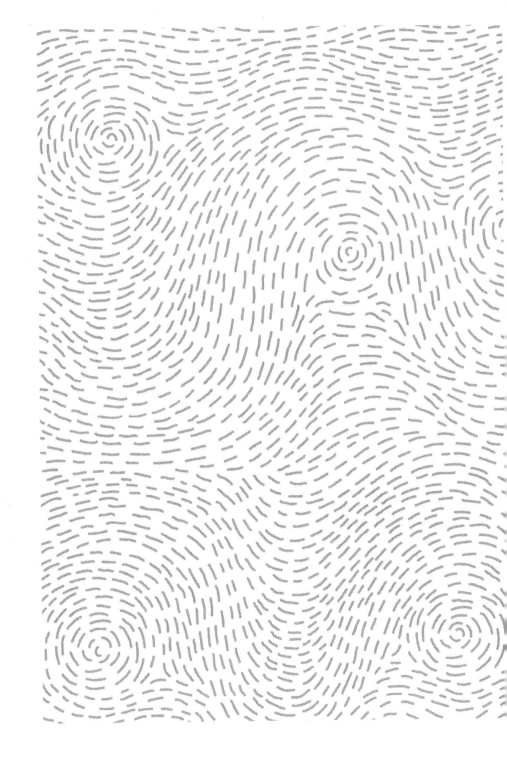

CHAPTER THREE

Make Your Own Green Smoothies

Whether you plan to enjoy green smoothies for breakfast, use them to replace unhealthy snacks, or drink them instead of eating fast-food for lunch or dinner, you'll find that they are very easy to make in just a few simple steps.

Before you get started, be sure you have selected a recipe and that you have all the ingredients you need. Peel, chop, and measure the vegetables and fruits you will be adding; it's a good idea to premeasure liquids, superfoods, spices, and other ingredients that you plan to use as well. This way, you'll have everything ready to add to the blender when it's time.

Start with a simple recipe that appeals to you, and be sure to taste a little bit of it before pouring a full serving into your glass. If you feel it needs a little more of a certain ingredient, go ahead and add what you want. Unlike recipes for cooking and baking that must often be followed exactly for good results, green smoothie recipes have plenty of room for variation. Making smoothies that taste great is the best way to encourage yourself to keep drinking them.

HOW TO MAKE GREEN SMOOTHIES FROM SCRATCH

After buying your ingredients, washing them, peeling them if needed, and cutting them into easily managed pieces, you're ready to make smoothies. The following steps will reduce wear and tear on your blender while ultimately creating drinks with a smooth, creamy texture.

Step One: Begin with Liquid

Liquid prevents vegetables and fruits from sticking to your blender's blade, particularly if you are using an inexpensive model. You can use water if you like, or you can use another liquid that appeals to you. The recipes in this book call for a variety of liquids, ranging from almond milk to flavored herbal tea. Once you are familiar with the flavors these liquids impart, you may want to start improvising to personalize your smoothies.

The amount of liquid you will need will vary, depending on your blender. Start with the amount a recipe recommends, and add a little more if you notice your blender is having difficulty processing the produce you are adding. When using additional liquid, add it a little at a time for best results.

Step Two: Add Thick or Creamy Ingredients

To prevent your smoothie from taking on a pulpy, mushy texture, add the thickest, creamiest ingredients next. To make things easy for you, the recipes contained in this book list ingredients in the order they should be added for best results. If you're making a recipe from another source or creating your own recipe, add things like banana, mango, papaya, pear, apple, peach, apricot, or avocado after placing liquid in the blender's reservoir.

If you are using nut butter, coconut meat, raw nuts, or seeds, add them during this step. In addition, if you are using any frozen ingredients or have premade a smoothie and are reconstituting it from frozen cubes, add frozen items after the liquid to keep them from sticking beneath the blades and damaging your blender's motor.

Step Three: Blend

Blend on high speed until the thick ingredients have been thoroughly incorporated with the liquid. If there are any lumps, blend a little longer. The amount of time required for the initial blending varies from one blender to the next, and some ingredients take longer to blend than others.

If you are using frozen ingredients, you may need to blend a bit longer. You may find that you need to pulse a few times for between three and five seconds before the blender will run easily. This depends on the blender;

some models have an "ice crushing" setting you can use to make the process a bit faster.

Step Four: Add Watery Fruits and Vegetables

Berries, melon, pineapple, citrus fruits, tomatoes, bell peppers, celery, and other watery fruits and vegetables are next to go into the blender. If you are making a single smoothie, you can probably add them all at once. If you are making a large batch, you may need to add about one cup at a time.

Step Five: Pulse

Using the "pulse" function on your blender, pulse for three to five seconds, then pulse again for five to ten seconds. Pulse a third time for ten seconds or so, and pulse again if your recipe still has large chunks. Keep pulsing until all the ingredients are well incorporated but not perfectly smooth.

Step Six: Incorporate Greens, Protein Powders, and Other Additives

Unless you have a very powerful blender, chop or tear your greens into pieces about an inch square before adding them to the blender. This will prevent lumpiness and bitterness, and it will also make the task of processing easier on your blender.

If you are adding protein powder, spirulina, or other boosts, do so during this step.

Step Seven: Pulse and Blend

After adding greens, pulse a few times for about three seconds each time. Next, either hit the "smoothie" button on your blender, or if there is none, blend on high speed. Allow the blender to run for thirty to sixty seconds, until you can see that there are no more chunks. If you notice that certain chunks just won't seem to blend, it could be that you've gotten a tough bit of fiber, such as a piece of apple core or pineapple core, into your recipe. You can either ignore it while sipping your smoothie, or you can use a spoon to fish it out of your glass.

Step Eight: Enjoy

Pour your smoothie into a glass, garnish it if you like, and proceed to enjoy it. Smoothies are often too thick to drink without a straw, so make sure you have straws on hand. If you prefer not to use disposable straws, you can find stainless steel straws online and in some kitchen supply stores. These are very easy to clean and sterilize, plus they add visual appeal.

GUIDELINES FOR ROTATING YOUR GREENS

Perhaps there are certain greens you like more than others. While you can enjoy these frequently, it is important to incorporate a variety of leafy green vegetables into your smoothie regimen. This promotes more complete nutrition, since not all greens contain the same nutrients or phytonutrients.

The second reason to use a variety of leafy greens and rotate them regularly is that all green leaves contain slight amounts of natural toxins, such as oxalic acid and goitrogens, that are there to deter predators from eating them. This does not mean that kale, spinach, or bok choy are poisonous; it simply means you should enjoy a mix of different greens throughout the week to prevent any natural toxins from building up in your body.

Different Plant Families, Different Toxins

Different plant families contain different types of toxins, so it is important to switch not just from one type of leafy green vegetable to another, but from one plant family to the next. There are four plant families that contain leafy greens:

- **Apiaceae:** Parsley and cilantro
- **Asteraceae:** All types of leaf lettuce, dandelion, and romaine lettuce
- **Amaranthaceae/Chenopodiaceae:** Beets, chard, lamb's-quarters, and spinach
- **Brassicaceae/Cruciferae:** Arugula, bok choy, broccoli, cabbage, collards, kale, mustard greens, and radish greens

There is no need to make your way through plants from all of these families during the course of a single week, unless you prefer to do so. Many people who enjoy green smoothies daily pick two types of greens from different families to use over the course of three days to a week, until their supply dwindles. Then they choose two types of greens from the remaining two families to use for the next few days. This ensures that plenty of nutrients make their way into the body, and it prevents the potential for overexposure to natural plant toxins.

Don't worry—rotating your greens will not hamper your ability to enjoy all the recipes in this book. If you'd like to try a certain recipe but the leafy greens it calls for are not in your current rotation, simply substitute the greens you are using for those in the recipe. Take the flavor of the greens into consideration when doing this. For example, a recipe that calls for Bibb lettuce will also work well with baby spinach, but it is not likely to work well with mustard greens. Adding more fruit or using fewer leafy greens are two very easy ways to ensure the flavors in your smoothie please your palate.

Besides finding smoothies with flavors you will enjoy, look for recipes that best suit your nutritional needs. If you need to lose weight, for example, use high-fat ingredients sparingly. If you have diabetes, be sure you are following the nutritional plan your doctor has recommended. By creating a plan that conforms to your needs, you will reap as many benefits as you possibly can.

FINDING THE RIGHT COMBINATIONS FOR YOU

Everyone has their own favorite flavors, and while this is a positive thing, most of us eventually find ourselves feeling bored when we have foods with the same few flavors over and over again. The recipes in this book have been carefully created to make sure most people will enjoy them. If you dislike certain fruits or if they are not available in your area, there is no need to use them. If you'd like to use an ingredient that is not listed in a recipe, feel free to give it a try.

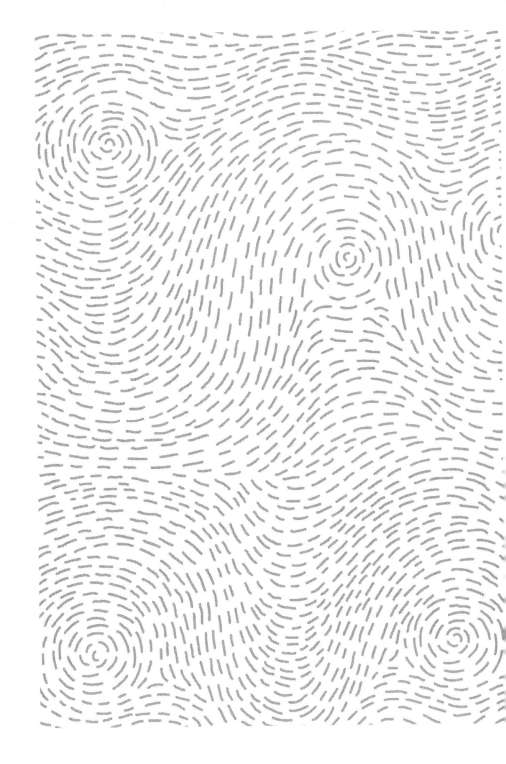

CHAPTER FOUR

Spice It Up

Once you are ready to create new recipes of your own, let your imagination run wild, but do look for inspiration. Food companies have conducted extensive (and expensive!) research to determine which flavor combinations people find most appealing, and these flavor combinations are everywhere—from commercially available juice blends to flavored yogurts.

While basic green smoothies are undeniably delicious, there are many ingredients you can add that will spice up your smoothie and take it to a whole new level.

TASTY INGREDIENTS TO ADD TO SMOOTHIES

Some of the recipes in this book contain herbs, spices, and other flavoring ingredients, including some of the following. But there are many others as well that you might like to try adding to your favorite smoothies.

Anise

Anise has a lovely licorice taste. It is ideal for enjoying in fruit smoothies.

Basil

Fresh basil has a distinct, unique aroma. It is perfect for incorporating into savory all-vegetable smoothies.

Cayenne Pepper

Cayenne pepper is known for its hot, spicy flavor. Unless you love very hot spices, start with just a pinch. Cayenne is excellent in smoothies that contain no fruit. It stimulates digestion and blood circulation, and consuming it can help you cool down rapidly when you are overheated.

Celery Seed

Celery seed has a fairly intense taste that is similar to fresh celery. Use a spice mill to grind it into a fine powder for best results.

Chipotle Chili

Chipotle imparts a warm, spicy taste to vegetable smoothies. It is not as intense as some other types of chilies, but comes with some of the same metabolic benefits.

Cilantro

Cilantro has a bright, clean, refreshing taste. It is delicious in vegetable smoothies. Note that many people have a distinct aversion or sensitivity to cilantro. Even if you love cilantro, your child or partner may think it tastes like soap. Test this wonderful herb out before you commit to using it in a smoothie.

Cinnamon

Cinnamon may help boost metabolism, and it gives a warm, delicious flavor to foods. A small amount of powdered cinnamon is great in a smoothie.

Cloves

Ground cloves have high levels of antioxidants and can be useful in reducing gastrointestinal symptoms such as diarrhea, nausea, and flatulence. This spice tastes wonderful when combined with other warm, sweet seasonings such as nutmeg, cinnamon, and ginger. A little pinch goes a long way.

Dill

Dill has a bright, pleasant flavor that makes green vegetable smoothies come to life. Fresh dill is best, but a pinch of dried dill leaves can be used as a substitute.

Garlic

Garlic offers numerous health benefits, and it tastes wonderful, too. While some people enjoy the taste of garlic only in vegetable smoothies, others find that they like it in smoothies that contain fruit as well.

Ginger

Gingerroot is very popular in juicing recipes, but it is extremely fibrous and not normally suitable for smoothies. Fresh ginger paste is available in some areas, as is powdered gingerroot. Both of these forms of the spice are excellent for smoothies.

Horseradish

Horseradish has a hot, intense flavor that can help clear the sinuses. It does not work well in fruit smoothies, but it tastes delicious with vegetables, especially tomatoes.

Mint

Mint has a delightfully refreshing flavor and a wonderful aroma. While it is often used as a garnish due to its bright green color and attractive leaves, it is an excellent addition to almost any green smoothie.

Mustard Powder

Prepared mustard gets much of its flavor from dried mustard powder, which has a distinct taste many people enjoy. This is an excellent spice to try in vegetable smoothies.

Nutmeg

While large amounts of nutmeg can be toxic and taste overpowering, a pinch of this warm, fragrant spice is delicious sprinkled on top of a smoothie or blended in with fruits such as apples or pears.

Rosemary

Rosemary is a wonderfully savory herb that enhances the taste of vegetable-only smoothies. Use fresh or powdered rosemary; dried whole leaves do not blend well.

Turmeric

Turmeric has a bright yellow color and a warm, interesting taste. It supports the digestive, immune, and cardiovascular systems and may aid in weight management.

Vanilla

Pure vanilla extract or vanilla bean concentrate are delicious in a wide variety of fruit smoothies. As little as a quarter teaspoon is enough to lend character to recipes, although some people enjoy the flavor so much that they use even more. Be sure to avoid artificial vanilla flavor and other artificial flavorings; they contain chemicals that do nothing to enhance your well-being.

Wasabi

Like horseradish, wasabi has a very intense, distinct flavor. This hot, savory spice is excellent in vegetable smoothies.

As toxins leave the body, they often contribute to headaches. Some spices help relieve those headaches. If you notice a headache coming on, try a smoothie made with ginger or cayenne pepper for natural relief.

SUPER SMOOTHIES: SUPERFOODS AND THEIR HEALTH BENEFITS

Specialty shops that offer green smoothies often charge high prices for drinks that have been boosted with superfoods. But there's no need to leave home to enjoy the benefits these concentrated nutrient sources provide. You can add these superfoods and others to nearly any smoothie without changing its taste dramatically. Be sure to follow package directions regarding serving size.

Açai Juice

Fresh açai berries are impossible to come by in most places, but minimally processed juice is often readily available. This juice has an intense flavor and is brimming with antioxidants. It is also an excellent source of anthocyanins, which contribute to heart health.

Blue-Green Algae

Blue-green algae has a less intense taste than kelp and other sea vegetables do, so if you'd like to reap the benefits while continuing to enjoy the flavor of smoothies that contain fruit, try adding half a teaspoon to a sixteen-ounce smoothie. Once you become accustomed to the taste, gradually work your way up to as much as two tablespoons of blue-green algae per serving.

Camu Powder

Camu powder contains plenty of vitamin C and is renowned for its ability to help ward off viruses like the common cold, while helping to improve skin tone and texture. It has a tart taste that combines well with fruits. Add about a teaspoon to a sixteen-ounce smoothie for a tasty boost.

Chia Seeds

Chia seeds contain the omega fatty acids your body requires for healthy brain function, plus they have been proven to help fight high cholesterol and contribute to heart health. These recipes recommend soaking the seeds in water prior to making the drink. Chia seeds become gelatinous when soaked this way, which helps your body to absorb their nutrients, and aids in digestion. Use up to three tablespoons of soaked fiber-rich chia seeds per sixteen-ounce smoothie.

Chlorella

Chlorella is a bright-green algae that is high in iron, betacarotene, and vitamin B_{12}. It is an excellent supplement for vegetarians and vegans. Use one teaspoon of chlorella per sixteen-ounce smoothie to enjoy its many benefits.

Cacao Nibs and Cocoa Powder

Cacao nibs are pieces of cacao beans that have been roasted and hulled—basically, raw chocolate. They are crunchy and taste somewhat similar to roasted coffee beans. Cacao nibs and cocoa powder give smoothies a tempting chocolate flavor that can help eliminate cravings. They also contain powerful flavonoids that can help keep blood sugar under control, along with antioxidants, vitamins, and minerals that support good health. The benefits of eating dark chocolate have been thoroughly documented, so be sure to add a few teaspoons of cocoa to your smoothies every now and then.

Coconut Oil

Organic coconut oil contains high levels of healthy fatty acids that can boost metabolism. Use up to a tablespoon of coconut oil per sixteen-ounce green smoothie.

Cranberry Juice

Cranberry juice is very high in vitamin C, and it contains plenty of antioxidants; it contributes just the right amount of tartness to smoothies. Be sure to buy pure cranberry juice with no added sugar or artificial sweeteners.

Flaxseed

Ground flaxseed is an excellent vegan source of essential omega-3 fatty acids, and it can also be used to make smoothies a little thicker. Use one tablespoon of ground flaxseed per sixteen-ounce smoothie.

Goji Berries

Dried goji berries contain more than twenty vitamins and minerals, as well as amino acids and antioxidants. Add half a cup to smoothies to sweeten them and give yourself a nutritional boost.

Hemp Protein

Hemp protein has more fiber than soy protein does, and it contains high levels of essential amino acids. Use between one and four tablespoons of hemp protein per sixteen-ounce smoothie.

Kelp and Other Sea Vegetables

Sea vegetables contain high levels of protein, vitamin A, iron, calcium, and other essential minerals. They can help to protect the immune system while adding an interesting flavor to vegetable smoothies. Powdered sea vegetables have a strong flavor that doesn't complement fruit well; use half a teaspoon to one tablespoon in green smoothies that contain vegetables only.

Maca Powder

Maca powder contains high levels of vitamins and minerals, including plenty of potassium. It also provides an energy boost. With a flavor that might remind you a bit of butterscotch, it is wonderful with mild-tasting fruits. Use up to two tablespoons per sixteen-ounce smoothie.

Moringa

Moringa contains high levels of antioxidants as well as plenty of vitamins and minerals. Derived from a flowering plant native to India, this superfood has a light, refreshing taste. Use one teaspoon of moringa powder in any sixteen-ounce smoothie.

Nuts

Nuts add caloric value to smoothies, plus they are an excellent source of protein and fiber that can add quite a bit of body to smoothies while providing a flavor boost. Raw almonds and cashews are fairly soft and are easy for most blenders to handle. Use about two tablespoons of nuts per sixteen-ounce smoothie.

Nut Butters

When choosing nut butters, be sure to select those that contain no additives such as high-fructose corn syrup, hydrogenated vegetable oil, or partially hydrogenated vegetable oil. These additives are empty calories and can have a detrimental effect on your well-being. Natural nut butters are available at most health food stores and even at some traditional supermarkets. Use one to two tablespoons per sixteen-ounce smoothie.

Pomegranate Juice

While you can add pomegranate seeds to your smoothie, they can be hard on your blender. A splash of pomegranate juice adds tartness while increasing your smoothie's antioxidant content.

Protein Powder

Protein stabilizes blood sugar and helps keep you feeling full. There are a wide variety of protein powders available. Choose one that appeals to you, but try to avoid artificial flavors because these can drastically alter the way your smoothies will taste.

Spirulina

Spirulina lends bright green color to smoothies while offering a boost of omega fatty acids and protein. Use between one and two teaspoons of spirulina in a sixteen-ounce smoothie to reap its rewards.

Wheat Germ

A good source of thiamin and vitamin E, wheat germ increases a smoothie's nutritional value without altering its flavor much at all. Use two tablespoons per sixteen-ounce smoothie.

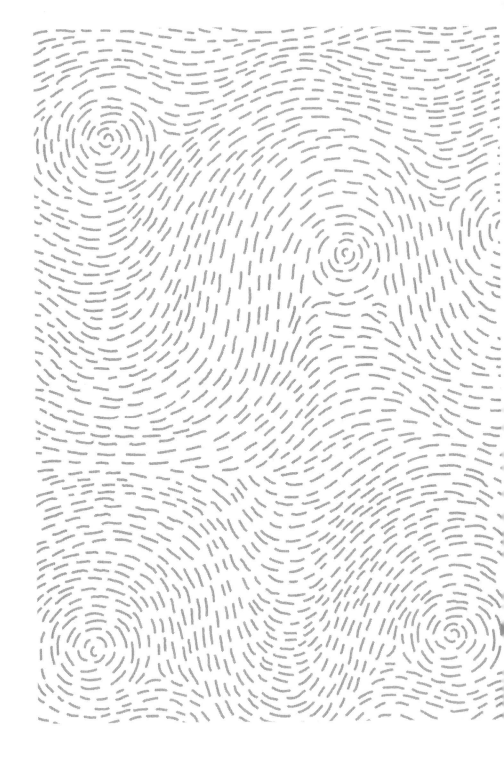

PART TWO

Green Smoothie Recipes

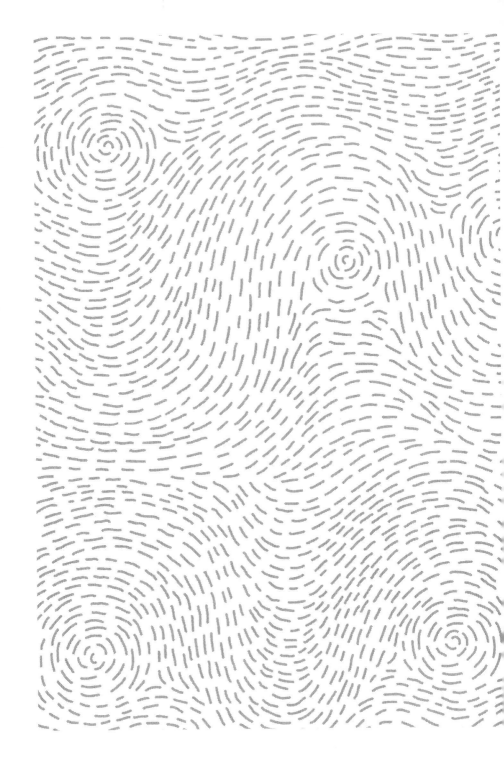

CHAPTER FIVE

Green Smoothies for Beginners

One of the best ways to get your veggies and fruits is to make delicious green smoothies at home. These are among the easiest and fastest foods to make, because they contain only a few ingredients and require minimal preparation. Each of the recipes in this chapter has been created with beginners in mind. All contain fruits and vegetables that are easy to find at most supermarkets or farmers markets, and none contain exotic ingredients or unfamiliar superfoods. All of them incorporate plenty of fruit, which will make it easy to introduce your palate to green smoothies.

As you prepare these recipes, remember to add the ingredients in the order listed and blend after each addition. This will give your smoothie the most appealing consistency. If you feel the smoothie should be thicker, add a few ice cubes after processing all the vegetables and fruits, and then blend them in until the mixture is once again smooth. Ice cubes can also help to make the flavors milder.

If you have never had a green smoothie before, you might be surprised at some of the incredible colors you'll soon see in your glass. Some are bright and beautiful, while others have decidedly unappetizing hues that can be somewhat off-putting to the uninitiated. It's not uncommon for beginning smoothie makers to find it difficult to convince themselves to go ahead and try the first recipe they make. If your smoothies look unappealing to you, pour them into opaque cups or glasses so you won't be able to see what you are drinking. Once you taste these delicious recipes, it's quite likely the green color will no longer bother you.

Banana-Berry Blast

YIELDS 2 CUPS

Bananas make an excellent addition to many sweet smoothies, lending a creamy texture and a pleasing taste to recipes of all kinds. They're perfect for enjoying pre- or postworkout, too, since they contain plenty of potassium. Strawberries are high in antioxidants and other nutrients; 1 cup contains 136 percent of the recommended daily allowance of vitamin C.

1 CUP WATER

1 BANANA, PEELED AND CUT INTO 1-INCH CHUNKS

1 CUP STRAWBERRIES, HULLED AND HALVED

1 CUP BABY SPINACH, LOOSELY PACKED

Blend all ingredients together, adding more liquid if the mixture is too thick. Pour your smoothie into a glass and enjoy immediately. If you'd like to add even more fruit flavor while increasing your vitamin C intake, replace the water with fresh citrus juice.

Bananas are often said to grow on trees, but these large plants are actually herbs. The sweet fruits are among the most popular in the world, with the average American consuming approximately 28 pounds of bananas annually. Unfortunately, if you are allergic to latex, you may also be allergic to bananas. Almost half of all people who are allergic to latex cannot enjoy bananas.

Mango Magic

Known as the "king of fruits," mangoes are among the most nutritious of all tropical fruits. With smooth, sweet, bright-orange flesh that has a buttery consistency, these delicious fruits provide potassium, betacarotene, vitamin A, alphacarotene, vitamin C, and other essential nutrients in abundance. Though low in calories, Bibb lettuce contains plenty of vitamins and minerals, along with potassium and folate.

1 CUP WATER
1 MANGO, PEELED, SEEDED, AND CUT INTO 1-INCH CHUNKS
½ CUP CHOPPED BIBB LETTUCE

Blend all ingredients together. Pour into a glass and enjoy immediately. For a more substantial smoothie, add half a banana or a splash of almond milk.

Perfect Pear

Ripe pears are wonderfully sweet while being low in calories and high in dietary fiber. They are a good source of minerals including manganese, magnesium, potassium, iron, and copper, along with B-complex vitamins including riboflavin and folate. The alfalfa sprouts provide protein while hiding among the other ingredients. If you're terrified of trying green smoothies, this recipe makes one that is barely green at all.

1 CUP WATER

1 PEAR, CORED AND CUT INTO CHUNKS

½ BANANA, PEELED AND CUT INTO 1-INCH CHUNKS

¼ TEASPOON PUMPKIN PIE SPICE

¼ TEASPOON PURE VANILLA EXTRACT

1 CUP ALFALFA SPROUTS

Blend all ingredients together, adding more water if the mixture is too thick. Pour into a glass and enjoy immediately. If you love the flavor of pears, add a second pear to the blender instead of the banana. If this combination tastes bland, add half a teaspoon of cinnamon along with the banana.

Tropical Tango

YIELDS 3 CUPS

Many people are surprised to discover that pineapples are actually very large berries. With forbidding, prickly exteriors and sweet, sunny-yellow flesh, they are a favorite green smoothie ingredient, thanks to their ability to deliver high doses of vitamin C, vitamin B_1, and potassium, along with many other essential nutrients. Romaine lettuce is wonderfully nutritious, but it has very little flavor, so it's easy to disguise. Smoothies that contain it often taste as though they have no greens in them at all.

1 CUP WATER

1 BANANA, PEELED AND CUT INTO 1-INCH CHUNKS

1 CUP PINEAPPLE, CUT INTO CHUNKS

½ CUP CHOPPED ROMAINE LETTUCE

Blend all ingredients together, adding more water if the mixture seems too thick. Pour into a glass and enjoy immediately. Use frozen pineapple chunks in place of fresh pineapple for a quick, cool treat, or add six to eight ice cubes to the blender after processing the rest of the ingredients.

Just Peachy

Peaches are popular because they are sweet, juicy, and intensely flavorful. While they are a delectable addition to green smoothies, they are also a good source of minerals, including iron and potassium, along with fluoride, which is necessary for strong bones and healthy teeth. They also contain plenty of antioxidants and essential vitamins.

1 CUP WATER

1 BANANA, PEELED AND CUT INTO 1-INCH CHUNKS

3 PEACHES, PITTED AND QUARTERED

3-INCH CUCUMBER SEGMENT, UNPEELED, WELL WASHED, AND SLICED

Blend all ingredients together, adding more water if the mixture is too thick. Pour into a glass and enjoy the smooth, delicious taste of fresh summer fruit. Feel free to use frozen peaches instead of fresh ones— they contain the same healthy fiber and offer the same delicious sun-ripened flavor.

Raspberry Delight

Raspberries are among the most nutritious of all the world's fruits, offering many essential vitamins including vitamin E, vitamin A, and vitamin C, which is a powerful antioxidant. Raspberries also contain high levels of iron and other minerals, including copper, which is essential for the formation of healthy red blood cells. Baby bok choy has a delicate flavor that virtually disappears in smoothies, yet it contains high levels of vitamins, minerals, and antioxidants.

1 CUP WATER

1 BANANA, PEELED AND CUT INTO 1-INCH CHUNKS

1½ CUPS RASPBERRIES

1 CUP CHOPPED BABY BOK CHOY, LOOSELY PACKED

Blend all ingredients together, starting with a little less liquid if you'd like to finish up with a thicker smoothie. Pour into a glass and enjoy. If raspberries are unavailable, try using blackberries instead. This recipe also works very well with frozen mixed berries; be sure to buy a brand with no added sugar.

Crazy for Coconut

YIELDS 3 CUPS

If you think of coconut as thin, sweetened shreds of sugary goodness, you've got the processed type in mind. Whole coconuts are filled with nutrient-rich water that has a light taste and plenty of electrolytes. Unsweetened coconut meat contains fiber and protein, as well as healthy monounsaturated fat. The pineapple in this recipe sweetens the coconut while adding tropical flair and disguising the light "green" flavor of the baby spinach.

1 CUP COCONUT WATER

1 CUP PINEAPPLE, CUT INTO CHUNKS

½ CUP UNSWEETENED COCONUT MEAT

1 CUP BABY SPINACH, LOOSELY PACKED

Blend all ingredients together, using less coconut water at the outset if you'd like a thicker, creamier smoothie. Pour into a glass and enjoy. Increase your protein intake by adding a quarter cup of raw cashews to this decadent smoothie.

Cool Citrus Greenie

YIELDS 3 CUPS

Fresh citrus fruit is rich in vitamins and minerals, and is cholesterol free, fat free, and sodium free. It contains the vitamins, minerals, and antioxidants your body needs for good health, and it provides a serious dose of dietary fiber. Kale is among the most nutritious of all leafy greens, offering an abundance of iron and other minerals, vitamins, and antioxidants.

1 CUP WATER

1 BANANA, PEELED AND CUT INTO 1-INCH CHUNKS

1 ORANGE, PEELED AND SEEDED

4 TANGERINES, PEELED AND SEEDED

½ CUP CHOPPED KALE

Blend all ingredients together, beginning with about half a cup of water and adding more as you go, if needed. Pour into a glass, garnish with a citrus wedge, and enjoy. For an even brighter taste, try using half a mango or a cup of pineapple in place of the banana.

Tangerines are also known as mandarin oranges or satsumas, and are sometimes marketed as special citrus fruits just for kids because they are small and easy to peel. Tangerines have a sweet, intense taste that many people find irresistible. Weighing in at just about 27 calories apiece, these appealing little fruits are valuable sources of antioxidants, plus they contain both soluble and insoluble fiber. If you're feeling tired, bored, or a bit blue, you can try peeling a tangerine and breathing its fragrance. The essential oil the skin contains has a wonderfully uplifting effect that can banish a bad mood.

Strawberry Sorbet

YIELDS 4 CUPS

Bright red with a sweet, irresistible flavor, fresh strawberries contain high levels of phytochemicals including ellagic acid and anthocyanins, both of which may aid in slowing the aging process and halting the progress of inflammation. High in vitamin C and B-complex vitamins, as well as vitamin A and vitamin E, strawberries also contain important minerals including iodine, copper, and iron.

1 CUP WATER

1 BANANA, PEELED AND CUT INTO 1-INCH CHUNKS

2 CUPS STRAWBERRIES, HULLED AND HALVED

3-INCH CUCUMBER SEGMENT, UNPEELED, WELL WASHED, AND SLICED

Blend all ingredients together, then pour into a glass and enjoy the taste of sun-ripened berries and smooth bananas. Try using frozen strawberries for a sweet, invigorating summertime treat you can enjoy anytime—even on winter's coldest mornings. For an even more delightful treat, try adding a quarter teaspoon of pure vanilla extract; it will give your smoothie a taste that's similar to fresh strawberry ice cream.

Blueberry Pie

Though nutrient-dense, both blueberries and blackberries are low in calories. Both contain high levels of antioxidants, vitamins, and minerals. Among these nutrients are chlorogenic acid, which aids in controlling blood glucose levels; lutein, which is vital for eye health; and B-complex vitamins, which aid in healthy metabolism.

1 CUP WATER

1 BANANA, PEELED AND CUT INTO 1-INCH CHUNKS

1 CUP BLUEBERRIES

1 CUP BLACKBERRIES

1 CUP BABY SPINACH, LOOSELY PACKED

Blend all ingredients together, starting with about half the water and adding the remainder a little at a time to get the consistency you desire. Pour your smoothie into a tall glass, sprinkle a few extra berries on top, and enjoy. To increase flavor and treat yourself to even more healthy antioxidants, try using pure blueberry juice in place of the water.

Grape Cooler

YIELDS 5 CUPS

Kale is an outstanding source of the mineral manganese, which is necessary for building strong bones and supporting the body's connective tissue. It also contains plenty of fiber, as do grapes, apples, and avocados—all of which play supporting roles in making this green smoothie wonderfully delicious.

1 CUP WATER

1 BANANA, PEELED AND CUT INTO 1-INCH CHUNKS

1 APPLE, CORED AND CUT INTO 1-INCH CHUNKS

½ AVOCADO, PEELED, SEEDED, AND CHOPPED

2 CUPS GREEN GRAPES

1 CUP CHOPPED KALE

Blend all ingredients together, beginning with about half the water and adding more as you go, if needed. Pour your smoothie into a glass and enjoy its green goodness. If you'd like to add even more fruit flavor while increasing your vitamin C intake, replace the water with fresh citrus juice.

CHAPTER SIX

Breakfast Smoothies

If you're not eating breakfast, you are probably not working as well as you could all day. If you have a tendency to skip breakfast to save time or calories, or even to get just a little more sleep, your brain and body are missing out, and you will be more likely to overeat later in the day to compensate. While fresh smoothies are always preferable, you can prepare these recipes the night before, so you can still enjoy those last few minutes of precious shut-eye without sacrificing your health.

You will benefit most from a breakfast that includes protein and plenty of fiber, along with a little bit of healthy fat, since this combination helps satisfy hunger, fuels the thought processes, keeps metabolism on an even keel, and helps you feel full until lunchtime. These breakfast smoothies aren't just delicious; they contain filling, robust ingredients that taste great and increase your energy level. In addition, these recipes are easy to double for sharing.

Feel free to make substitutions. For example, if you have a nut allergy, you can use another type of milk in place of the nut milks many of these recipes call for, and you can replace nut butters with other filling ingredients such as avocado or the protein powder of your choice.

Granola in a Glass

YIELDS 3 CUPS

Oats contain high levels of essential omega-3 fatty acids, along with plenty of folate, potassium, and fiber, while almonds contain heart-healthy mono-unsaturated fat. The pure maple syrup in this recipe contains zinc, which is an important antioxidant.

1½ CUPS ALMOND MILK

½ BANANA, PEELED AND CUT INTO 1-INCH CHUNKS

1 APPLE, CORED AND CUT INTO CHUNKS

½ CUP ROLLED OATS

¼ CUP RAW ALMONDS

½ CUP BABY SPINACH, LOOSELY PACKED

1 TEASPOON MAPLE SYRUP

Blend all ingredients together, adding a little more almond milk if you feel the mixture is too thick. Pour into a glass and enjoy. Try replacing the apple with a pear for a milder taste. If you don't have maple syrup on hand, you can use a quarter teaspoon of cinnamon or a pinch of nutmeg to add flavor.

Almonds truly are a superfood, offering a complete, balanced source of energy and important nutrients. They are particularly rich in monounsaturated fats that increase HDL (good) cholesterol while reducing LDL (bad) cholesterol. In addition, almonds contain a high level of vitamin E, along with riboflavin, niacin, folate, and vitamin B_6. They are also high in important minerals, including potassium, manganese, iron, calcium, and selenium. Eating one handful of almonds each day is a good way to provide your body with many of the nutrients—and much of the protein—that it needs.

Wheat Germ Wake-Up

YIELDS 2 CUPS

Wheat germ is high in protein, antioxidants, vitamins, and minerals. It also promotes healthy digestion while providing the energy you need to get you through even the most challenging mornings. The sweetness of the banana tempers the bright, tart flavor of the orange.

1 CUP GREEN TEA, CHILLED

1 BANANA, PEELED AND CUT INTO 1-INCH CHUNKS

2 ORANGES, PEELED AND SEEDED

1 CUP CHOPPED BABY BOK CHOY, LOOSELY PACKED

1 TABLESPOON WHEAT GERM

Blend all ingredients together, adding more green tea if you feel that the mixture is too thick. Pour into a tall glass and enjoy. Transform this breakfast smoothie by replacing the oranges with other fruits. Strawberries, blueberries, pineapple, and mangoes are all excellent with bananas.

Peanut Butter Cookie

YIELDS 2 CUPS

Peanut butter is high in protein and contains just the right amount of fat to keep you feeling full all morning. The almond milk in this recipe is also high in protein, and the bananas provide plenty of sweetness to please your palate.

1½ CUPS UNSWEETENED ALMOND MILK

1 BANANA, PEELED AND CUT INTO 1-INCH CHUNKS

2 TABLESPOONS PEANUT BUTTER

2 TABLESPOONS ROLLED OATS OR WHEAT GERM

1 CELERY STALK, LONG FIBERS REMOVED, CHOPPED

Blend all ingredients together, beginning with about half a cup of almond milk and gradually adding more, as you like. Spoon or pour your smoothie into a glass and enjoy the comforting taste of nutritious peanut butter. When shopping for ingredients, look for all-natural peanut butter without any unhealthy hydrogenated or partially hydrogenated fats. Though natural peanut butter needs to be refrigerated and must be stirred before using, it is much better for your body.

Mango-Pineapple Sunshine

YIELDS 3 CUPS

While mango and pineapple contain an abundance of antioxidants, vitamins, minerals, and fiber, honey is more than just a sweetener. In addition to simple sugars, this golden liquid contains minerals, vitamins, protein, and enzymes that help metabolize cholesterol. Buying local honey supports beekeepers in your area.

1 CUP FRESH ORANGE JUICE

1 CUP FROZEN MANGO CHUNKS

1 CUP FROZEN PINEAPPLE CHUNKS

1 TABLESPOON LOCAL HONEY

3-INCH CUCUMBER SEGMENT, UNPEELED, WELL WASHED, AND SLICED

Blend all ingredients together, adding a little water or more orange juice if the consistency seems too thick. Pour into a glass and enjoy. This is a light, refreshing breakfast that's perfect for savoring on a warm summer morning—or even a cold winter day when you're wishing the sun would return. Add protein powder for a more filling finished product.

Berry Basket Breakfast

YIELDS 3 CUPS

Though this recipe has a delightfully refreshing taste, it is very satisfying, thanks to the fiber in the oatmeal and the protein in the almond milk. The Greek yogurt provides a pleasant tang, and the banana adds just the right amount of sweetness while providing plenty of potassium.

1 CUP ALMOND MILK

¼ CUP GREEK YOGURT

1 BANANA, PEELED AND CUT INTO 1-INCH CHUNKS

1 CUP STRAWBERRIES, HULLED AND HALVED

½ CUP BLACKBERRIES

1 CUP CHOPPED ROMAINE LETTUCE, LOOSELY PACKED

Blend all ingredients together, adding a little more almond milk or some water if you feel the mixture is too thick. Pour the finished product into a glass and savor the flavor of tart berries and delicious yogurt. If you're in the mood for a chilly treat, try using frozen banana chunks and frozen berries in place of fresh ones.

Toast and Jam

YIELDS 3 CUPS

Wheat germ and oatmeal offer a pleasant whole-grain taste, while straw-berries provide your taste buds with a tart, sweet wake-up call. This filling smoothie offers plenty of fiber and protein to keep you feeling energetic, and thanks to the strawberries, it also contains high levels of antioxidants.

1 CUP UNSWEETENED ALMOND MILK

½ BANANA, PEELED AND CUT INTO 1-INCH CHUNKS

1 CUP STRAWBERRIES, HULLED AND HALVED

1 TABLESPOON ROLLED OATS

1 TABLESPOON WHEAT GERM

3-INCH CUCUMBER SEGMENT, UNPEELED, WELL WASHED, AND SLICED

1 TEASPOON LOCAL HONEY

¼ TEASPOON PURE VANILLA EXTRACT

Blend all ingredients together, adding more almond milk if it is becoming too thick for the blender to handle. Spoon or pour this thick, creamy smoothie into a glass and enjoy. If you'd like to add even more fruit flavor while increasing your antioxidant intake, try using half a cup of blueberries or raspberries in place of the banana. This recipe works very well with frozen berry blends, too. If you decide to use frozen berries, be sure to choose those with no added sugar.

Pomegranate Protein

YIELDS 3 CUPS

Like red wine and green tea, pure pomegranate juice contains plenty of the antioxidants your body needs to help ward off cellular damage. Choose an organic brand if possible, and be sure it has no added sugar. The protein in the nuts and almond milk in this breakfast smoothie will power you through your morning.

1 CUP PURE POMEGRANATE JUICE

¾ CUP UNSWEETENED ALMOND MILK

1 BANANA, PEELED AND CUT INTO 1-INCH CHUNKS

2 TABLESPOONS RAW OR BLANCHED ALMONDS, ROUGHLY CHOPPED

1 TABLESPOON LOCAL HONEY

1 CUP BABY SPINACH, LOOSELY PACKED

Blend all ingredients together, beginning with half of the pomegranate juice, adding the remainder when you incorporate the almonds. Spoon or pour into a glass and enjoy. If you'd like to add even more protein to this delicious pomegranate smoothie, add 2 tablespoons of your favorite protein powder.

While you can eat pomegranate seeds or add them to a smoothie, the most convenient way to enjoy the many benefits this dark red fruit provides is to purchase commercially produced pomegranate juice that contains no added sugar, preservatives, or other impurities. Pomegranate has no fat or cholesterol, and it contains ellagitannin compounds, including punicalagin and granatin B, which researchers believe may be effective in reducing the risk of heart disease. Regular consumption of pomegranate has shown to be effective against diabetes, lymphoma, and other conditions.

Banana Crunch

YIELDS 2 CUPS

Top a green smoothie with your favorite granola for an even more satisfying breakfast. If you're pressed for time and prefer to enjoy your smoothies while commuting, place your granola in a small reusable container and munch it between sips.

1 CUP ALMOND MILK

1 BANANA, PEELED AND CUT INTO 1-INCH CHUNKS

1 TABLESPOON LOCAL HONEY

½ CUP CHOPPED BUTTER LETTUCE, LOOSELY PACKED

½ CUP GRANOLA

Blend all ingredients together except the granola and pour in a glass, leaving room for the cereal. For a thicker smoothie minus the crunch, blend the granola into the smoothie; if you do this, you may need a little more almond milk. When shopping for granola, look for a brand that contains all-natural ingredients.

Sunrise Surprise

YIELDS 3 CUPS

While whole almonds are high in calories and fat, unsweetened almond milk contains just about 40 calories per cup, and it provides plenty of calcium, vitamin D, vitamin E, and protein. It makes an excellent addition to green smoothies because it has a mild, pleasant taste that blends well with other flavors. If you don't like almond milk, feel free to use dairy milk, soy milk, or another type of nut milk in these recipes.

1 CUP ALMOND MILK

½ CUP PINEAPPLE, CUT INTO CHUNKS

2 PEACHES, PITTED AND QUARTERED

1 CUP STRAWBERRIES, HULLED AND HALVED

½ CUP CHOPPED KALE, LOOSELY PACKED

Blend all ingredients together, beginning with half of the almond milk and gradually adding more to the blender as you incorporate the fruit. Pour into a glass and enjoy. When preparing kale for your smoothie, cut the leaves away from the central ribs. This keeps out much of the bitterness that's so often associated with kale.

Fast Track Freeze

YIELDS 3 CUPS

Yogurt contains active cultures called probiotics, which aid in healthy digestion. Greek yogurt is thicker, richer, and higher in protein than traditional yogurt. This nutritious dairy product is also rich in calcium and phosphorous, both of which are important for building a strong, healthy body. If you do not eat dairy products, substitute nondairy yogurt and nut milk or soy milk for the skim milk and Greek yogurt in this recipe.

1 CUP SKIM MILK

½ CUP NONFAT GREEK YOGURT

1 BANANA, PEELED AND CUT INTO 1-INCH CHUNKS

1 CUP FROZEN BLUEBERRIES

1 TABLESPOON LOCAL HONEY

1 CUP BABY SPINACH, LOOSELY PACKED

Blend all ingredients together, adding a bit more skim milk if you feel the consistency is too thick. Pour into your favorite travel mug and enjoy. For an icier experience, use frozen banana chunks or add six to eight ice cubes to the blender after incorporating the spinach.

Tofu Temptation

Tofu lends creamy texture and pleasing body to smoothies. Packed with healthy protein and containing just a little fat, it combines well with nearly everything. When shopping for tofu, be sure to choose a brand made with soy that has not been genetically modified.

1 CUP WATER

½ CUP SOFT TOFU, DRAINED AND CUT INTO CUBES

1 BANANA, PEELED AND CUT INTO 1-INCH CHUNKS

½ CUP STRAWBERRIES, HULLED AND HALVED

½ CUP MANGO, PEELED, SEEDED, AND CUT INTO CHUNKS

½ CUP CHOPPED BABY BOK CHOY, LOOSELY PACKED

Blend all ingredients together, adding a little more water if the mixture is too thick. Spoon or pour the finished smoothie into a glass and enjoy this delicious meal replacement. If you'd like to add even more fruit flavor while increasing your vitamin C intake, replace the water with fresh citrus juice.

CHAPTER SEVEN

Super Green (Fruit-Free) Smoothies

If you're trying to end a sugar addiction or if you are on a diet that requires you to limit or eliminate all sugars—even those in fruit—you'll love these super green smoothies.

When making smoothies that contain no fruit, you may miss the creamy texture that bananas, mangoes, and other rich fruits impart. By adding avocado, you can regain that creamy consistency without drastically changing the flavors of the recipes you make. While not all of the recipes in this chapter call for avocado, you can certainly add it if you like.

Another way to enhance fruit-free smoothies is by combining herbs with the greens to lend savory flavor. When you are changing the way you eat, you may notice that you miss some of your favorite foods. Adding fresh herbs will help you to satisfy cravings without creating any feelings of guilt.

Finally, when making super green smoothies, consider using flavored herbal teas, lemon juice, lime juice, and stevia to impart a zesty flavor without increasing calorie content dramatically. In addition, consider adding a bit of extra ice to smoothies if the "green" taste is a little too strong for your palate at first.

Broccoli Salad

While broccoli is extremely low in calories, it contains high levels of vitamin C, which is a powerful immune booster and antioxidant—helping to ward off viruses, including the dreaded common cold. It also contains an abundance of folate, vitamin A, and B-complex vitamins, along with a small amount of omega-3 fatty acids.

1 CUP WATER

½ AVOCADO, PEELED, SEEDED, AND CHOPPED

1 CUP BROCCOLI FLORETS

1 CUP CHOPPED KALE

2 TABLESPOONS FRESH PARSLEY, CHOPPED

8 ICE CUBES

Blend all ingredients together, adding more water if the consistency is too thick for your blender to handle with ease. Pour into a glass and enjoy. If you find the flavor of this green smoothie to be too bland, try adding a teaspoon of fresh lemon juice or a dash of your favorite hot sauce.

Swiss Splendor

YIELDS 2 CUPS

Sometimes referred to as silverbeet, Swiss chard is a member of the beet family that is native to the Mediterranean region. This delicious leafy green is an excellent source of numerous nutrients, including vitamin K, which is essential for strong, sturdy bones. People who eat Swiss chard regularly are at lower risk for osteoporosis, vitamin A deficiency, and iron-deficiency anemia.

1 CUP WATER

½ AVOCADO, PEELED, SEEDED, AND CHOPPED

1 CUP CHOPPED SWISS CHARD

1 CUP BABY SPINACH, LOOSELY PACKED

1 TABLESPOON FRESH LIME JUICE

Blend all ingredients together, beginning with about half a cup of water and gradually adding more if needed. Pour into a glass and enjoy. If the tart taste of this smoothie is too much for you, add a small amount of natural stevia extract to sweeten it.

Salad in a Glass

YIELDS 2 CUPS

With a complete medley of vegetables, including leaf lettuce, baby spinach, tomato, cucumber, and carrot, plus tasty additions that include onion, fresh parsley, and zingy lemon juice, this liquid salad recipe sounds a bit odd but is wonderfully delicious. It's very low in calories, so you can enjoy as much as you like while treating your body to an abundance of vitamins and minerals.

1 CUP WATER

1 CUP CHOPPED GREEN OR RED LEAF LETTUCE

1 CUP BABY SPINACH, LOOSELY PACKED

1 TOMATO, CHOPPED

3-INCH CUCUMBER SEGMENT, UNPEELED, WELL WASHED, AND SLICED

1 CARROT, PEELED AND SLICED THINLY

1 SMALL SLICE ONION

1 TABLESPOON FRESH PARSLEY, CHOPPED

1 TEASPOON FRESH LEMON JUICE

Blend all ingredients together, adding more water if you feel the mixture is becoming too thick. Pour into a glass and savor the smoothie's taste and aroma. If you dislike onion, feel free to leave it out. To transform this recipe's flavor, try using different herbs in place of the parsley. Some fresh options to try include basil, cilantro, chives, or rosemary.

Spicy Salsa

Jalapeño peppers contain an alkaloid compound called capsaicin, which imparts their spicy, pungent flavor. Rich in vitamin C, which aids in the formation of collagen within the body, this smoothie also contains high levels of vitamin K and vitamin A, along with vitamin E and numerous beneficial flavonoids that help to protect the body's cells from disease.

1 CUP WATER

2 VINE-RIPENED TOMATOES, CHOPPED

¼ TO ½ JALAPEÑO, SEEDED, DERIBBED, AND CHOPPED

¼ CUP CILANTRO, CHOPPED

1 GREEN, RED, OR YELLOW BELL PEPPER, SEEDED,
    DERIBBED, AND CHOPPED

1 TEASPOON FRESH GARLIC, CHOPPED

1 CUP CHOPPED RED OR GREEN LEAF LETTUCE

1 TEASPOON FRESH LIME JUICE

Blend all ingredients together. Leave the lid on the blender for about 30 seconds after stopping the blade to allow microscopic particles of jalapeño to settle; skipping this step can lead to respiratory upset and eye pain. Pour into a glass and enjoy. If you dislike hot spices, try this recipe without the jalapeño; the flavor is milder, but is still fantastic.

* *

If you like the idea of trying jalapeño peppers in your green smoothies, be sure to remove the seeds and veins from the peppers before tossing them into the blender. These portions of the plant are hottest. Handle jalapeños and other hot peppers with care; many professionals wear kitchen gloves when dealing with them, as oils can transfer to skin and remain there even after you've washed your hands. Finally, if you've consumed a too-hot jalapeño, don't try to quench the heat with water; drink milk or another protein-rich beverage instead, because that's what neutralizes the capsaicin.

Italian Garden

YIELDS 2 CUPS

Zucchini is surprisingly high in protein, antioxidants, and potassium, yet it is extremely low in calories. The tomatoes in this recipe are high in lycopene and other antioxidants, and the fresh garlic also contains antioxidants that may lower cholesterol for improved heart health. This delicious green smoothie has a distinctive Italian flavor.

1 CUP WATER

6-INCH ZUCCHINI SEGMENT, CHOPPED

1 TEASPOON MINCED FRESH GARLIC

2 VINE-RIPENED TOMATOES, CHOPPED

2 TABLESPOONS FRESH BASIL, CHOPPED

2 CUPS CHOPPED ROMAINE LETTUCE, LOOSELY PACKED

Blend all ingredients together, adding more water if you feel the mixture is becoming too thick. Pour into a glass and enjoy. Adjust the amount of garlic you use to please your palate; if you find the taste of fresh garlic to be overpowering, use half a teaspoon to begin with. If, on the other hand, you love the flavor of garlic, add as much as you like.

Minty Fresh

YIELDS 2 CUPS

Mint leaves might be low in calories, but they offer an abundance of fiber, along with a considerable amount of vitamin A. Like other herbs, fresh mint allows you to flavor foods without additional sodium or seasonings laced with chemicals. Cucumbers are very low in calories, though they are highly nutritious.

1 CUP MINT TEA, CHILLED

1 CUP CHOPPED ROMAINE LETTUCE, LOOSELY PACKED

3-INCH CUCUMBER SEGMENT, UNPEELED, WELL WASHED, AND SLICED

2 TABLESPOONS CHOPPED FRESH MINT

8 ICE CUBES

Blend all ingredients together, beginning with just half of the mint tea and adding the rest as you incorporate the remainder of the ingredients. Pour into a glass and enjoy. If you'd like to add sweetness to this recipe, you can add a few drops of natural stevia extract.

Mixed Green Medley

YIELDS 2 CUPS

Whether you are on a low-carbohydrate diet or you're simply looking after your health, you will enjoy the many wonderful benefits that fresh, leafy green vegetables provide. Dark leafy greens are an excellent source of vitamins and minerals, and they contain small amounts of omega-3 fatty acids as well. Though this green smoothie is very low in calories, it delivers a bonanza of essential nutrients.

1 CUP WATER
1 CUP CHOPPED KALE, LOOSELY PACKED
1 CUP BABY SPINACH, LOOSELY PACKED
1 CUP CHOPPED SWISS CHARD, LOOSELY PACKED
1 CUCUMBER, UNPEELED, WELL WASHED, AND SLICED
1 TABLESPOON FRESH LEMON JUICE
8 ICE CUBES

Blend all ingredients together, adding more water or a little more lemon juice if you feel the mixture is becoming too thick. Pour into a glass and enjoy. You can transform this recipe by using flavored herbal tea instead of water and eliminating the lemon juice. You can also add a bit of natural stevia extract or honey to infuse your smoothie with natural sweetness.

Zesty Tomato Toss-Up

YIELDS 2 CUPS

Although tomatoes are found in the vegetable aisle at the market, these sweet, fragrant members of the nightshade family are actually fruits. Containing an average of just 16 calories, a medium-size vine-ripened tomato contains no fat or cholesterol. And though it is a fruit, it is also low in sugar. Tomatoes contain a number of important nutrients, including flavonoids, antioxidants, minerals, and vitamins.

1 CUP WATER

¼ AVOCADO, PEELED AND SEEDED

3 VINE-RIPENED TOMATOES, CHOPPED

3-INCH CUCUMBER SEGMENT, UNPEELED, WELL WASHED, AND SLICED

1 TABLESPOON FRESH PARSLEY, CHOPPED

1 CUP CHOPPED KALE, LOOSELY PACKED

2 STALKS CELERY, LONG FIBERS REMOVED, CHOPPED

Blend all ingredients together, adding a little more water if needed. Pour into a tall glass and enjoy the smooth, lightly sweet taste of refreshing veggies. For even more flavor, try adding more herbs, including fresh basil or rosemary, or some garlic. If you enjoy the taste of sage or oregano, feel free to try these herbs. Use sparingly, though, as they can overpower other flavors.

There are many varieties of tomatoes, with some of the most flavorful being known collectively as heirloom tomatoes. These old-fashioned tomatoes come in a vast array of colors, ranging from yellow to dark purple, and they offer superior flavor as well as interesting nutritional profiles. As interest in heirloom tomatoes grows, they are becoming easier to find at farmers markets and even in some supermarkets. Unlike hybrid tomatoes, they are usually found only during the summer months—their natural growing season.

Beet Chiller

YIELDS 2 CUPS

Vibrant purple beets are valuable both for their colorful roots and their nutritious green leaves. Closely related to Swiss chard, these earthy vegetables are an excellent source of B vitamins and minerals, including iron, copper, manganese, and magnesium. Beets are also a very good source of potassium, which lowers heart rate while regulating metabolism at a cellular level.

1 CUP WATER

1 BEET, PEELED AND CUT INTO ½-INCH CHUNKS

1 CARROT, PEELED AND SLICED THINLY

1 CUCUMBER, UNPEELED, WELL WASHED, AND SLICED

2 STALKS CELERY, LONG FIBERS REMOVED, CHOPPED

1 CUP CHOPPED BABY BOK CHOY

6 ICE CUBES

Blend all ingredients together, adding more water if needed, then pour into a glass and enjoy. To minimize staining on your hands, peel the beet under running water or wear a pair of protective food-grade gloves. Protect your cutting board from the beet's bright red juice by covering it with parchment paper.

Cucumber Cooler

YIELDS 2 CUPS

Low in calories, bursting with pure, delicious water, and overflowing with potassium, vitamins, minerals, and antioxidants, cucumbers are also mild diuretics, which means they help release excess water weight from the body while easing the burden of high blood pressure. Celery adds a lightly salty flavor to this recipe, while baby spinach provides many important vitamins and minerals, including an abundance of iron.

1 CUP WATER
1 CUCUMBER, UNPEELED, WELL WASHED, AND SLICED
2 STALKS CELERY, LONG FIBERS REMOVED, CHOPPED
1 CUP BABY SPINACH, LOOSELY PACKED
6 ICE CUBES

Blend all ingredients together, adding more water if it is becoming too thick, then pour into a glass and enjoy. This super-simple green smoothie has a very light, pleasant flavor and is just right for rehydrating on a hot, humid day.

Bell Pepper Blast

YIELDS 2 CUPS

Often referred to as sweet peppers, bell peppers are not normally spicy at all. In fact, red, orange, and yellow bell peppers often have a very sweet taste that makes them perfect for adding to smoothies of all kinds. Despite their sweet taste, they are very low in calories. Fresh bell peppers contain an abundance of antioxidants, too, including vitamin A and vitamin C; they also contain plenty of essential minerals and B-complex vitamins.

1 CUP WATER

1 GREEN BELL PEPPER, SEEDED, DERIBBED, AND CUT INTO
    1-INCH CHUNKS

1 YELLOW BELL PEPPER, SEEDED, DERIBBED, AND CUT INTO
    1-INCH CHUNKS

1 STALK CELERY, LONG FIBERS REMOVED, CHOPPED

3-INCH CUCUMBER SEGMENT, UNPEELED, WELL WASHED, AND SLICED

1 CUP CHOPPED ROMAINE LETTUCE

1 TABLESPOON CILANTRO, CHOPPED

1 TABLESPOON FRESH LEMON OR LIME JUICE

Blend all ingredients together, adding more water if you feel the mixture is too thick, then pour into a glass and enjoy. If you'd like to add even more flavor and you enjoy hot spices, try adding a pinch of cayenne pepper. The capsaicin it contains may help rev up your metabolism.

CHAPTER EIGHT

Smoothies for Weight Loss

Losing weight can be difficult, and though people often blame a lack of willpower for plateaus and regained pounds, sometimes the problem is that many are seriously undernourished when following weight-loss diets. When you replace unhealthy snacks and meals with green smoothies, even if it's just once or twice a day, you will discover that excess pounds seem to melt away without drastically altering your diet.

The nutrients these powerful smoothies contain ensure that your body's cells are able to function at an optimal level, even though you are taking in fewer calories. As a result, you keep on burning energy rapidly. On a standard weight-loss diet that simply relies on reduced caloric intake, the lack of proper nutrition can cause the body to believe it is starving. When that happens, you burn calories at a greatly reduced pace. This metabolic process is deeply ingrained in our DNA; long ago, when food was often scarce, our bodies learned to conserve calories during lean times.

The recipes in this chapter have been designed to help nourish your body while promoting feelings of fullness and satisfying cravings. Each contains protein as well as a small amount of healthy fat, plenty of fiber, and enough calories to prevent your metabolism from slowing. While these smoothies will help you manage your dietary intake and reset your taste buds so you crave healthy options rather than junk food, increasing your physical activity will help you lose weight even faster.

Chia Champion

YIELDS 3 CUPS

Chia seeds have been used as food since 3500 BCE. Once a staple of native people who inhabited the southwestern United States and Mexico, these little seeds provide concentrated calories and protein. A single tablespoon is packed with 2 grams of protein, 5 grams of carbohydrate, and a little over 3 grams of healthy monounsaturated and polyunsaturated fats. Soaking these seeds changes their texture and makes them easily digestible.

1 CUP GREEN TEA, CHILLED

1 BANANA, PEELED AND CUT INTO 1-INCH CHUNKS

1 CUP RASPBERRIES

2 TEASPOONS CHIA SEEDS, SOAKED IN WATER FOR 30 MINUTES

2 CUPS CHOPPED RED OR GREEN LEAF LETTUCE, LOOSELY PACKED

Blend all ingredients together, adding a little more tea if the mixture is too thick, then pour into a glass and enjoy. If you are avoiding caffeine, you can use filtered water or caffeine-free herbal tea to replace the green tea in this recipe.

Chia seeds contain an exceptionally high amount of calcium, with 3 tablespoons providing an incredible 233 milligrams of the bone-building nutrient. This is just a little less than the amount of calcium found in a cup of milk, which has 299 milligrams of calcium. In addition, chia seeds contain iron, zinc, magnesium, potassium, phosphorus, and other vital minerals.

Peach Power

Not only do peaches add their signature color to smoothies, they also provide a smorgasbord of vitamins, minerals, and other important nutrients. With just 40 calories per medium peach, these luscious little fruits contain a mere 9 grams of sugar, yet they taste as if they contain much more. This recipe also incorporates nutritious mangoes and protein-rich almond milk, along with mild-tasting baby bok choy.

1 CUP UNSWEETENED ALMOND MILK

1 MANGO, PEELED, SEEDED, AND CUT INTO 1-INCH CHUNKS

1 PEACH, PITTED AND QUARTERED

1 CUP CHOPPED BABY BOK CHOY

Blend all ingredients together, adding a little more almond milk if the mixture is thicker than you'd like it to be, then pour into your favorite glass and enjoy. This recipe is fantastic with frozen fruit or fresh.

Minty Melon

YIELDS 2 CUPS

Honeydew melon has a light, sweet taste and a consistency that's somewhat like cantaloupe. This delicious fruit provides a significant amount of vitamins and minerals, along with a healthy helping of antioxidants. The alfalfa sprouts in this recipe contain a high level of protein that will provide you with a feeling of satisfaction.

1 CUP PEPPERMINT TEA, CHILLED

1 CUP HONEYDEW MELON, PARED, SEEDED, AND CUT INTO CHUNKS

3-INCH CUCUMBER SEGMENT, UNPEELED, WELL WASHED, AND SLICED

½ CUP ALFALFA SPROUTS

1 CUP CHOPPED BUTTER LETTUCE

Blend all ingredients together, adding more peppermint tea if you'd like a thinner consistency. Pour into a glass and enjoy. For additional mint flavor, add 2 tablespoons of fresh mint leaves to the recipe. If you prefer a sweeter smoothie, add a few drops of natural stevia extract.

Melon Madness

Romaine lettuce is the perfect green for light-tasting smoothies. With a very mild flavor and just 106 calories in an entire head, it is 17 percent protein and contains all 8 essential amino acids. This refreshing lettuce is also high in omega-3 fatty acids, iron, vitamin C, and vitamin A, and it contains plenty of essential minerals.

1 CUP WATER

1 CUP HONEYDEW MELON, PARED, SEEDED, AND CUT INTO CHUNKS

1 CUP CANTALOUPE, PARED, SEEDED, AND CUT INTO CHUNKS

2 TEASPOONS CHIA SEEDS, SOAKED FOR 30 MINUTES

2 CUPS CHOPPED ROMAINE LETTUCE

Blend all ingredients together, adding more water if you prefer a thinner consistency. Pour into a glass and enjoy. If you are craving an icy blended smoothie, freeze your melon chunks before adding them.

Watermelon Slush

YIELDS 2 CUPS

Abundant during the hot summer months, watermelon is a wonderfully hydrating fruit that offers plenty of potassium, betacarotene, and lycopene. Seedless watermelons are easy to eat, but they are often less flavorful than those with seeds. Since watermelon seeds are very high in protein, and they are pulverized when blended, they make a valuable addition to smoothies.

1 CUP WATER OR HERBAL TEA, CHILLED

2 CUPS WATERMELON, CUT INTO CHUNKS

½ CUCUMBER, UNPEELED, WELL WASHED, AND SLICED

2 TEASPOONS CHIA SEEDS, SOAKED FOR 30 MINUTES

4 ICE CUBES

Blend all ingredients together, pour into a glass, and enjoy a fantastic summertime treat. This recipe is great for showcasing the flavor of any melon. Simply replace the watermelon with honeydew melon or cantaloupe for a refreshing, low-calorie treat.

Berry-Vanilla Chiller

Vanilla beans are actually seed pods obtained from tropical climbing orchids that open for one day only; they typically must be pollinated by hand to ensure crop survival. Pure vanilla extract contains small amounts of B-complex vitamins that aid in nervous system function and regulating metabolism. Vanilla extract may be added to almost any fruit-flavored smoothie. It adds a luscious aroma and a delicious taste.

1 CUP ALMOND MILK

2 CUPS FROZEN BLUEBERRIES

1 TABLESPOON FLAXSEED, SOAKED IN WATER FOR 30 MINUTES

1 TEASPOON PURE VANILLA EXTRACT

1 CUP CHOPPED BABY BOK CHOY

Blend all ingredients together, beginning with about half a cup of almond milk and adding more after the blueberries have been incorporated. Pour into a glass and enjoy. If you prefer, make this recipe with frozen strawberries or a frozen berry blend. When shopping, be sure to select frozen berries with no added sugar.

Berries Galore

Alfalfa sprouts are marvelous on sandwiches and salads, and they make a wonderful addition to green smoothies, too. Easy to grow in a jar on your kitchen counter, these delicious sprouts contain only 12 calories per cup, yet they are rich in vitamin A, vitamin C, vitamin B, vitamin B_{12}, and vitamin K. They have also been shown to fight inflammation and reduce cholesterol.

1 CUP BERRY-FLAVORED HERBAL TEA, CHILLED

1 CUP RASPBERRIES

1 CUP STRAWBERRIES, HULLED AND HALVED

1 CUP ALFALFA SPROUTS

Blend all ingredients together, pour into a glass, and enjoy. If the berry flavor is a little too intense for you, add four to six ice cubes to the blender after adding the alfalfa sprouts.

Alfalfa sprouts can be expensive at the supermarket, and they can spoil quickly, too. If you like the taste, consider growing your own. All you need are organic alfalfa seeds and a simple alfalfa sprout growing kit, which consists of a series of screened lids that fit atop a standard canning jar. Growing your own greens is simple and convenient, and it will save you money.

Berries and Cream

YIELDS 3 CUPS

While fresh fruits are delicious, frozen fruits are usually picked at the peak of ripeness, then flash-frozen and packaged for sale. These fruits contain the same nutrition as fresh ones, so don't hesitate to stock up and use them in your green smoothies.

1 CUP SKIM MILK

1 CUP FROZEN RASPBERRIES

1 CUP FROZEN BLUEBERRIES

1 SCOOP VANILLA-FLAVORED PROTEIN POWDER

¼ TEASPOON PURE VANILLA EXTRACT

3-INCH CUCUMBER SEGMENT, UNPEELED, WELL WASHED, AND SLICED

NATURAL STEVIA EXTRACT FOR SWEETENING

Blend all ingredients together, adding more milk if the mixture is thicker than you'd like it to be. Pour into a glass for immediate satisfaction. If you are avoi-ding dairy products, you can use soy milk or your favorite nut milk in place of the skim milk.

Berry Abundant

YIELDS 4 CUPS

Blackberries grow wild in many places; in fact, they are so abundant in some areas that they are considered to be a nuisance. If possible, consider harvesting some of these berries for your smoothies. They taste fantastic and are brimming with vitamins, minerals, and antioxidants. If you have a garden, think about growing your own berries. You'll save money on smoothie ingredients and you'll never have to wonder how your berries were handled.

1 CUP SKIM MILK

¼ AVOCADO, PEELED AND SEEDED

1 CUP BLACKBERRIES

1 CUP STRAWBERRIES, HULLED AND HALVED

1 CUP RASPBERRIES

2 TEASPOONS FLAXSEED, SOAKED IN WATER FOR 30 MINUTES

1 CUP BABY SPINACH, LOOSELY PACKED

Blend all ingredients together, pour into a glass, and enjoy. This is a fantastic recipe to share with someone who might be reluctant to try green smoothies. It has a rich, creamy taste with just the right amount of berry flavor. Add a little extra sweetness with natural stevia extract, if you like.

Mango-Apricot Parfait

YIELDS 2 CUPS

Mangoes offer numerous health benefits. While they are higher in sugar and calories than some other fruits, they offer plenty of fiber, potassium, and vitamin C. In addition, they are rich in carotenoids, which are fat-soluble antioxidants that protect the brain and nervous system while guarding against high cholesterol and heart disease. The almond milk in this simple recipe adds protein, while the lettuce adds valuable vitamins and minerals.

1 CUP ALMOND MILK

1 MANGO, PEELED, SEEDED, AND CUT INTO CHUNKS

2 APRICOTS, PITTED AND HALVED

1 CUP CHOPPED BUTTER LETTUCE

Blend all ingredients together, adjusting the amount of almond milk to suit your taste, then pour into a glass and enjoy. If fresh apricots are not available, you can achieve a similar taste and texture by using a fresh peach or nectarine. Frozen peach slices with no sugar added will do in a pinch.

Apple Pie à la Mode

YIELDS 2 CUPS

Apples contain high levels of antioxidants that can help keep sickness at bay, lending truth to the old saying "An apple a day keeps the doctor away." Low in calories with no fat or cholesterol, apples contain plenty of fiber, along with B-complex vitamins, and flavonoids such as quercetin, procyanidin B_2, and epicatechin. In addition, they contain important minerals that aid in healthy metabolism.

1 CUP SKIM MILK

1 APPLE, CORED AND CUT INTO CHUNKS

¼ TEASPOON PURE VANILLA EXTRACT

3-INCH CUCUMBER SEGMENT, UNPEELED, WELL WASHED, AND SLICED

½ TEASPOON CINNAMON

PINCH OF NUTMEG

NATURAL STEVIA EXTRACT FOR SWEETENING

Blend all ingredients together, pour into a glass, and enjoy. This is an excellent green smoothie to try if you are craving a fattening dessert. While it is very low in calories, it offers plenty of flavor, plus protein to satisfy your hunger.

CHAPTER NINE

Detox and Cleansing Smoothies

Toxic substances are all around us. The air we breathe is often polluted, the food we eat is frequently contaminated with heavy metals, and the water we drink has all kinds of chemicals, some of which have been added to make it "safe." Viruses, harmful bacteria, and other invaders frequently make their way onto or into our bodies; we consume them in our food, we pick them up when we touch items others have touched, and we breathe them in while sharing personal space.

Our bodies are capable of eliminating most harmful substances, but they need a little help. Green smoothies aid in the detoxification process by providing the body's cells with the antioxidants they need to eliminate toxins, repair themselves, and defend against future attacks. While it is undoubtedly beneficial to detox from time to time, the best course of action is to enjoy green smoothies regularly to keep our defenses strong—that way, there's less damage in the first place.

Whether you decide to cleanse and detoxify your body by undergoing a green smoothie fast that lasts a few days, or if you simply decide to drink detoxifying smoothies daily, you are likely to notice some side effects at first. These include headaches, diarrhea, skin rashes and outbreaks, and severe moodiness. Keep up your green smoothie habit, though, and all of these side effects will disappear within a few days, leaving you feeling better than you may have in quite some time.

Amazing Antioxidants

YIELDS 3 CUPS

Antioxidants are nutrients that slow or completely prevent the damage that occurs as our cells naturally produce free radicals after using oxygen. These metabolic by-products can lead to such problems as macular degeneration, diabetes, cancer, and heart disease. Antioxidants can enhance the body's immune response and reduce the risk that these problems, and similar ones, will occur.

1 CUP PURE POMEGRANATE JUICE

1 CUP SEEDLESS PURPLE GRAPES

1 CUP MIXED FROZEN BERRIES

1 CUP CHOPPED KALE, LOOSELY PACKED

Blend all ingredients together, pour into a glass, and enjoy. If the tart, tangy taste of this green smoothie is too strong for you, add a few drops of natural stevia extract for a bit of sweetness.

Carrot Cleanse

YIELDS 3 CUPS

*Carrots are naturally sweet, crunchy, and delicious. There are several differ-
ent types grown around the world, including some in interesting colors such
as purple, yellow, and red. Rich in antioxidants, vitamin A, and betacarotene,
they also contain flavonoid compounds that may aid in preventing lung, skin,
and oral cavity cancers.*

1 CUP FRESH CARROT JUICE

1 CUP FROZEN MANGO CHUNKS

1 CUP FROZEN PINEAPPLE CHUNKS

¼ CUP FRESH PARSLEY

Blend all ingredients together, pour into a glass, and enjoy. If you'd like
to add even more succulent fruit flavor while increasing this smoothie's
detoxifying effect, add the juice of half a lemon.

*There are several different cultivars of parsley, but all are suitable
for culinary use, and all contain powerful antioxidants and have a
rich, delicious fragrance. Parsley also contains numerous vitamins
and minerals, along with essential volatile oils such as eugenol,
which was traditionally used by dentists as a natural antiseptic
to ward off gum disease and tooth decay. Parsley is also renowned
for its high vitamin K content; of all known herbs, it is the highest,
containing 1,366 percent of the recommended daily intake per
100-gram serving.*

Green Apple

There are several varieties of collard greens grown throughout the world. These robust greens are low in calories, yet they contain high amounts of essential nutrients such as folate, vitamin K, and vitamin A.

1 CUP GREEN TEA, CHILLED

1 GRANNY SMITH APPLE, CORED AND CUT INTO CHUNKS

1 BANANA, PEELED AND CUT INTO 1-INCH CHUNKS

1 CUP CHOPPED COLLARD GREENS, LOOSELY PACKED

¼ CUP FRESH PARSLEY

Blend all ingredients together, pour into your favorite glass, and enjoy. This beautiful, bright-green smoothie is also delicious when made with frozen banana chunks and four to six ice cubes.

Tropical Splendor

YIELDS 3 CUPS

Herbal detox tea, also known as herbal cleansing tea, is available in a variety of appealing flavors. Look for it at health food stores and at some supermarkets, as well as from online retailers. Brew a large pot of the tea and store it in the refrigerator to use in smoothies. You can also make ice cubes with it to enhance your smoothie's texture while imparting additional cleansing power.

1 CUP HERBAL DETOX TEA, CHILLED

1 MANGO, PEELED, SEEDED, AND CUT INTO 1-INCH CHUNKS

1 CUP PAPAYA, PEELED, SEEDED AND CUT INTO CHUNKS

2 TABLESPOONS FRESH LIME JUICE

½ CUP CHOPPED COLLARD GREENS, LOOSELY PACKED

PINCH OF CAYENNE PEPPER

Blend all ingredients together, adding more tea if the mixture is too thick. Pour into a glass and enjoy. If you prefer a frosty treat, freeze the mango and papaya chunks. For a less intense taste and even more detoxifying power, make ice cubes with herbal detox tea; add four to six of them to your smoothie.

Collard greens are among the most powerful of all popular leafy green vegetables. They contain powerful phytonutrients with proven anticancer properties against breast, prostate, cervical, ovarian, and colon cancers. These nutrients include DIM (diindolylmethane) and sulforaphane, which inhibit cancer cell growth while having a cytotoxic effect on existing cancer cells. Folate, vitamin A, vitamin C, and numerous minerals are just a few of the additional nutrients this incredible plant contains.

Berry-Citrus Parfait

YIELDS 2 CUPS

Rich in vitamins, minerals, and important phytonutrients, cabbage is inexpensive and widely abundant. This humble plant also contains powerful antioxidants that are known to help protect against prostate, colon, and breast cancer while aiding in the reduction of LDL (bad) cholesterol. Fresh cabbage offers abundant vitamin C, along with B vitamins, minerals, and vitamin K.

1 CUP FRESH ORANGE JUICE
½ CUP FROZEN RASPBERRIES
½ CUP FROZEN BLUEBERRIES
1 TANGERINE, PEELED AND SEEDED
½ CUP CHOPPED CABBAGE, LOOSELY PACKED

Blend all ingredients together, adding more juice or some water if you'd like a thinner consistency. Pour into a glass and drink immediately. If cruciferous vegetables disagree with you, replace the cabbage in this recipe with any of your favorite greens. Kale, spinach, bok choy, and lettuce work very well in this recipe.

Pear Pleasure

Among the world's most popular fruits, pears provide plenty of vitamin C and 6 grams of fiber per serving, along with numerous other minerals, vitamins, and antioxidants. A medium pear contains an average of 100 calories.

1 CUP FRESH CARROT JUICE

1 PEAR, CORED AND CUT INTO 1-INCH CHUNKS

1 BEET, PEELED AND CHOPPED INTO ½-INCH CHUNKS

1 APPLE, CORED AND CUT INTO 1-INCH CHUNKS

¼ TEASPOON GINGER

1 CUP BABY SPINACH, LOOSELY PACKED

Blend all ingredients together, pour into a glass, and enjoy. If this blend isn't quite sweet enough for you, add a few drops of natural stevia extract or a small amount of local honey.

Cucumber Contentment

Offering a light taste that lends itself perfectly to chilling, honeydew melon has a pleasant, light-green color. It offers an abundance of vitamins and minerals, while the lime adds a little extra vitamin C and zesty flavor.

1 CUP GREEN TEA, CHILLED
½ CUCUMBER, UNPEELED, WELL WASHED, AND SLICED
2 CUPS HONEYDEW MELON, PARED, SEEDED, AND CUT INTO CHUNKS
JUICE FROM 1 LIME
2 TABLESPOONS FRESH MINT

Blend all ingredients together, pour into a glass, and savor the sweet, refreshing flavor of cucumber, fresh mint, and melon. Double or triple this recipe to share with friends. Its light green color is festive and attractive.

Kiwi Tangelo Tango

YIELDS 3 CUPS

Tangelos are bright orange citrus fruits that result from hybridizing tangerines and grapefruits. Very high in vitamin C, low in calories, and extremely juicy, they offer abundant B vitamins and folate, along with niacin, calcium, and magnesium. The kiwifruits increase the smoothie's vitamin C content, while the grapefruit juice adds lycopene, betacarotene, lutein, and other essential nutrients.

1 CUP FRESH RUBY RED GRAPEFRUIT JUICE

2 KIWIS, PEELED AND HALVED

3 TANGELOS, PEELED AND SEEDED

2½ TABLESPOONS DRIED GOJI BERRIES

½ CUP CHOPPED KALE, LOOSELY PACKED

Blend all ingredients together, pour into a glass, and enjoy. If tangelos are unavailable, replace with six tangerines or two navel oranges.

Often referred to as the "queen of greens," kale is a member of the Brassicaceae family, which includes cruciferous vegetables such as collards, Brussels sprouts, cabbage, and broccoli. One cup of chopped kale contains just 33 calories, yet it provides an average of 684 percent of the U.S. recommended daily value of vitamin K, 134 percent of the vitamin C the body needs each day, and numerous other nutrients, including powerful carotenoids and flavonoids that provide anticancer benefits. Kale also helps lower blood cholesterol, bind bile acids, and reduce the risk of heart disease. Do use caution if you take anticoagulants such as warfarin; the high level of vitamin K in kale can interfere with the drug's function.

Basil-Melon Purifier

YIELDS 4 CUPS

Known as the "king of herbs," basil contains high levels of phytonutrients known to have healthy and disease-fighting properties. Flavonoids, including the antioxidants vicenin and orientin, betacarotene, vitamin A, lutein, and vitamin K are just some of the nutrients this fragrant, tasty herb contains. While this recipe calls for only a small amount, you can certainly add more if you do not find the flavor to be overpowering.

1 CUP GREEN TEA, CHILLED

2 CUPS HONEYDEW MELON, PARED, SEEDED, AND CUT INTO CHUNKS

3-INCH CUCUMBER SEGMENT, UNPEELED, WELL WASHED, AND SLICED

1 CUP CHOPPED KALE, LOOSELY PACKED

JUICE FROM 1 LIME

4 LEAVES FRESH BASIL

8 ICE CUBES

Blend all ingredients together, pour into a glass, and enjoy. If you dislike the taste of basil, or if fresh basil isn't available, replace it with 2 tablespoons of fresh parsley.

Lean and Green

YIELDS 3 CUPS

This delicious smoothie is heavy on the greens, but it contains three large servings of fruit to provide balance. Some of its key nutrients include potassium, vitamin C, vitamin A, folate, lutein, and vitamin K. To increase the recipe's antioxidant power, use chilled green tea in place of water.

1 CUP WATER

1 BANANA, PEELED AND CUT INTO 1-INCH CHUNKS

1 CUP FROZEN PINEAPPLE CHUNKS

1 CUP FROZEN MANGO CHUNKS

JUICE FROM ½ LEMON

½ CUP BABY SPINACH, LOOSELY PACKED

½ CUP CHOPPED CABBAGE, LOOSELY PACKED

Blend all ingredients together, pour into a glass, and enjoy this smooth, delicious treat. If you prefer, you can transform this smoothie's flavor by using either 2 cups of frozen pineapple chunks or 2 cups of frozen mango chunks. Both options are delightful.

Different varieties of cabbage are widely cultivated around the world, and all are brimming with nutrition. Some types of cabbage you might encounter include mild-tasting Napa cabbage, vibrant red cabbage, and dark-green leafy cabbage; bok choy is also a member of the cabbage family. Cabbage contains numerous phytonutrients, including sulforaphane, xanthan, and thiocyanates. These antioxidants are known to aid in preventing cancer, plus they aid in reducing

LDL (bad) cholesterol. Some types of cabbage contain compounds called goitrogens, which can cause swelling of the thyroid gland in persons suffering from thyroid dysfunction. Talk to your doctor about the pros and cons of consuming large amounts of cabbage if you have thyroid disease.

Tropical Sensation

YIELDS 2 CUPS

Closely related to lemons, oranges, and other citrus fruits, the interesting flavor of lime is wonderfully refreshing. Limes are high in vitamin C, which is essential for connective tissue health and wound healing. Other nutrients in this smoothie include potassium, vitamin A, numerous amino acids, and an abundance of healthy fiber.

1 CUP COCONUT WATER

1 BANANA, PEELED AND CUT INTO 1-INCH CHUNKS

1 CUP HONEYDEW MELON, PARED, SEEDED, AND CUT INTO CHUNKS

½ CUP PINEAPPLE, CUT INTO CHUNKS

JUICE FROM ½ LIME

½ CUP CHOPPED BUTTER LETTUCE, LOOSELY PACKED

6 ICE CUBES

Blend all ingredients together, adding a little more coconut water if the finished product is too thick. Pour into a glass and enjoy. For an extra protein boost and a more intense coconut taste, add 2 tablespoons of unsweetened coconut meat to the blender along with the butter lettuce.

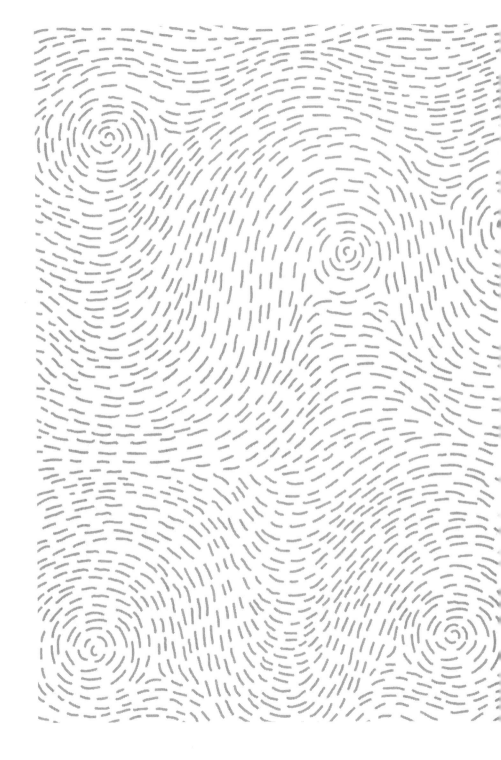

CHAPTER TEN

Smoothies for Digestive Health

Green smoothies can improve the body's ability to absorb nutrients properly, and can also aid in promoting overall gastrointestinal health. If you suffer from a digestive disorder or inflammatory bowel disease, constipation, celiac disease, or gastric reflux, you may find that drinking green smoothies regularly can help to ease your symptoms and may enable you to reduce or eliminate your dependence on prescription and over-the-counter medications for digestive issues.

Smoothies aid in healthy digestion because they are very easy for the body to assimilate. They give the digestive system a much-needed break and a chance to heal itself, particularly if you use them to replace unhealthy options. Just drinking one green smoothie daily can make a difference. In fact, it is important to ease your way into a green smoothie habit to give your digestive system a chance to become accustomed to the extra fiber and other nutrients smoothies contain. Consuming too much at once can lead to bloating and gas, particularly if you normally avoid foods that are high in fiber.

When adding protein to smoothies for digestive health, it's a good idea to choose fermented or nondairy options over cows' milk or goats' milk, since these can disrupt digestion. Whey-based protein powders can also aggravate digestive issues, because they can irritate the intestines and stomach lining. Better options are yogurt, kefir, and dairy-free yogurt containing live cultures. While some of the recipes in this chapter call for these ingredients, you can add them to any smoothie to increase your protein intake while improving your digestive health.

Apple-Ginger Parfait

YIELDS 2 CUPS

Ginger is a favorite traditional remedy for digestive upset, and the fiber in apples and baby bok choy can help soothe a turbulent tummy. If you have a very powerful blender, you can use a half-inch section of peeled fresh gingerroot in place of the powdered ginger. The taste will be a bit spicier, but the soothing effect will be more pronounced.

1 CUP WATER

1 APPLE, CORED AND CUT INTO 1-INCH CHUNKS

½ TEASPOON POWDERED GINGER

1 TABLESPOON LOCAL HONEY

½ CUP CHOPPED BABY BOK CHOY

6 ICE CUBES

Blend all ingredients together, beginning with half of the water and adding more as you incorporate the baby bok choy. When finished, pour into a glass and enjoy. Replace half of the water with an equal amount of soy milk, nut milk, or skim milk. This adds protein, and transforms this light, refreshing smoothie into a meal.

Chamomile Calmer

When gas disrupts your digestive system, bloating, discomfort, and embarrassment can result. The chamomile tea this recipe contains can help to release gas that is trapped in your digestive system. In addition, chamomile is a relaxing brew. The fiber in the apple and spinach aid digestion, while the parsley adds flavor and reduces bloating.

1 CUP CHAMOMILE TEA, CHILLED

1 APPLE, CORED AND CUT INTO 1-INCH CHUNKS

1 TABLESPOON FRESH PARSLEY

1 CUP BABY SPINACH, LOOSELY PACKED

Blend all ingredients together, then pour into a glass and enjoy this relaxing, refreshing beverage. If you don't have fresh parsley on hand, you can add ¼ teaspoon of ginger instead for added flavor. It will also help alleviate gastrointestinal discomfort.

Banana Tummy Tamer

YIELDS 2 CUPS

While all vegetables and fruits contain healthy fiber that can boost digestive health, bananas are easier to digest than some others. Try this simple smoothie when recovering from the flu or suffering from indigestion. It has a mild taste that won't induce nausea.

1 CUP WATER

2 BANANAS, PEELED AND CUT INTO 1-INCH CHUNKS

1 CUP CHOPPED BIBB LETTUCE, LOOSELY PACKED

Blend all ingredients together, pour into a glass, and enjoy. While this recipe works well with other greens, mild-tasting Bibb or butter lettuce won't irritate your stomach when you're not feeling your best.

Sometimes referred to as limestone lettuce, Bibb lettuce is a type of butterhead lettuce that has a delicate green taste. With just 7 calories per cup, Bibb lettuce contains high levels of vitamin A and vitamin K. It is also rich in folate and potassium. If you are growing a garden, consider planting a row or two of Bibb lettuce. This variety grows rapidly, even in cool weather, and can tolerate high temperatures. It takes about 43 days to mature and can be grown in containers or sown directly into soil.

Hydration, Please

YIELDS 4 CUPS

Of all the nutrients that are essential for good digestion, water is among the most important. Without it, food moves through the intestines too slowly, which can lead to gas and bloating. While all green smoothies are hydrating, this recipe contains more water than most others. It makes an excellent postworkout treat.

1 CUP WATER, CHILLED

2 CUPS HONEYDEW MELON, PARED, SEEDED, AND CUT INTO CHUNKS

2 CUPS CHOPPED GREEN LEAF LETTUCE, LOOSELY PACKED

6 ICE CUBES

Blend all ingredients together, pour into a tall glass, and enjoy this smoothie's light, refreshing flavor. If you like, you can freeze the honeydew melon chunks before adding them. Consider preparing and freezing an entire honeydew in advance so you can enjoy this smoothie any time you like.

Yes to Yogurt

YIELDS 2 CUPS

Yogurt that contains live cultures is an excellent addition to your diet, because these beneficial bacteria help to eliminate any bad bacteria that may be living in your digestive system. If you do not eat dairy products, use a dairy-free yogurt made with live cultures L. acidophilus *and* B. bifidum. *These are the same cultures dairy yogurt contains.*

1 CUP WATER

½ CUP PLAIN YOGURT

1 MANGO, PEELED, SEEDED, AND CUT INTO CHUNKS

1 CUP BABY SPINACH, LOOSELY PACKED

Blend all ingredients together, pour into a glass, and enjoy. Add a little more water if the smoothie is too thick, and incorporate a few ice cubes at the end if it's not thick enough. This recipe works very well with any fruit, including peaches, strawberries, papaya, and pineapple. If you find the flavor is too tart, add a few drops of natural stevia extract or up to 1 tablespoon of local honey for natural sweetness.

Oats and Berries

YIELDS 3 CUPS

Oatmeal contains a type of fiber known as prebiotics, which probiotics (good bacteria) feed on so they can multiply. Berries and Swiss chard also contain prebiotics, and the dietary fiber in all of these ingredients goes the extra mile by helping to lower the level of LDL (bad) cholesterol in your bloodstream while helping to keep blood sugar stable.

1 CUP WATER

1 BANANA, PEELED AND CUT INTO 1-INCH CHUNKS

½ CUP RASPBERRIES

½ CUP BLACKBERRIES

½ CUP STRAWBERRIES, HULLED AND HALVED

¼ CUP ROLLED OATS

½ CUP CHOPPED SWISS CHARD, LOOSELY PACKED

Blend all ingredients together, pour into a glass, and enjoy. If you'd like to add even more fruit flavor while increasing your vitamin C intake, replace the water with fresh citrus juice.

. . . .

Various Swiss chard varieties are typically available in spring, summer, and autumn, though growing seasons vary by area. With large, deep-green leaves and crisp, edible stems that are less bitter than those of many other leafy greens, chard contains numerous antioxidants, including vitamin A and vitamin C, plus an abundance of vitamin K, plenty of omega-3 fatty acids, folate, vitamin B₆, niacin, and essential minerals. Regular consumption of chard may help prevent osteoporosis and anemia, and may also aid in preventing cardiovascular disease and certain cancers, including prostate and colon cancer. If you are on an anticoagulant such as warfarin, chard can cause toxicity and should be avoided. In addition, chard contains oxalic acid, which can crystalize as oxalate stones in the urinary tracts of individuals who are prone to them.

Red Sunset

Beets and beet greens are rich in fiber, helping to keep waste moving through the small and large intestines. In addition, these foods contain lots of magnesium, potassium, iron, calcium, and betacarotene, all of which are essential to maintaining the health of the smooth muscles that line the digestive tract.

1 CUP FRESH ORANGE JUICE

1 BANANA, PEELED AND CUT INTO 1-INCH CHUNKS

1 BEET, PEELED AND CUT INTO ½-INCH CHUNKS

1 CUP STRAWBERRIES, HULLED AND HALVED

½ CUP CHOPPED BEET GREENS, INCLUDING STEMS

Blend all ingredients together, pour into a tall glass, and savor. For additional fruit flavor, add a peeled, seeded orange or tangerine to the blender along with the chopped beet.

Avocado Shake

YIELDS 3 CUPS

Avocados are excellent for digestive health. Not only does a medium fruit contain an incredible 15 grams of fiber, it also has a healthy dose of mono-unsaturated fat, which stimulates healthy functioning of the gall bladder, pancreas, and liver. This type of fat helps convert betacarotene into vitamin A, which is essential for building the gastrointestinal tract's mucosal lining.

1 CUP WATER

½ AVOCADO, PEELED, SEEDED, AND CHOPPED

1 BANANA, PEELED AND CUT INTO 1-INCH CHUNKS

2 CUPS HONEYDEW MELON, PARED, SEEDED, AND CUT INTO CHUNKS

1 CUP CHOPPED ROMAINE LETTUCE, LOOSELY PACKED

Blend all ingredients together, pour into a glass, and relish this smoothie's creamy, delectable goodness. For an even more decadent treat that's surprisingly good for you, freeze the banana and honeydew melon, and add ¼ teaspoon of pure vanilla extract to the blender.

Cantaloupe Cooler

YIELDS 4 CUPS

Cantaloupe contains high levels of vitamin C, vitamin A, folate, vitamin B_6, essential enzymes, and fiber that aids the digestive process. It also contains enzymes called superoxide dismutases, which aid in reducing inflammation and supporting cellular defense. This powerful food may be low in calories, but it still helps to build a healthy body.

1 CUP WATER

2 CUPS CANTALOUPE, PARED, SEEDED, AND CUT INTO CHUNKS

1 CUP STRAWBERRIES, HULLED AND HALVED

½ CUP ALFALFA SPROUTS

6 ICE CUBES

Blend all ingredients together, pour into a glass, and enjoy. If you don't like high-protein alfalfa sprouts, you can replace them with another green, such as leaf lettuce, cabbage, or baby bok choy.

Kiwi Kiss

YIELDS 2 CUPS

Bright green kiwifruit tastes marvelous, and is an excellent food for the digestive system. It contains high levels of pepsin, an essential enzyme used in breaking down protein for proper assimilation. It also contains potassium, magnesium, essential fatty acids, and plenty of vitamins, including vitamin C and vitamin E.

1 CUP WATER

1 BANANA, PEELED AND CUT INTO 1-INCH CHUNKS

¼ AVOCADO, PEELED AND SEEDED

3 KIWIS, PEELED AND HALVED

1 CUP BABY SPINACH, LOOSELY PACKED

Blend all ingredients together, pour into a glass, and enjoy. While milk can replace water in many recipes, this is not one of them. The pepsin in kiwis makes milk curdle.

Papaya Perfection

YIELDS 4 CUPS

Papaya isn't just a delicious tropical fruit; it is also excellent for digestive health. Its nutrient-rich flesh contains papain, a proteolytic enzyme that facilitates effective digestion. It also contains protease inhibitors, tannins, alkaloids, anthraquinones, and beneficial flavonoids, which combine to give it powerful antioxidant and anti-inflammatory properties. Finally, papaya has been shown to lower triglycerides and serum cholesterol counts—all excellent reasons to enjoy it as often as you like.

1 CUP WATER

1 BANANA, PEELED AND CUT INTO 1-INCH CHUNKS

2 CUPS PAPAYA, PEELED, SEEDED, AND CUT INTO CHUNKS

½ CUP PINEAPPLE, CUT INTO CHUNKS

1 CUP BABY SPINACH, LOOSELY PACKED

Blend all ingredients together, pour into a glass, and enjoy. For a wonderfully delicious iced treat, use frozen fruit chunks. Papaya has been known to cause allergic reactions in some individuals. Be sure that you are not one of them before consuming it in green smoothies.

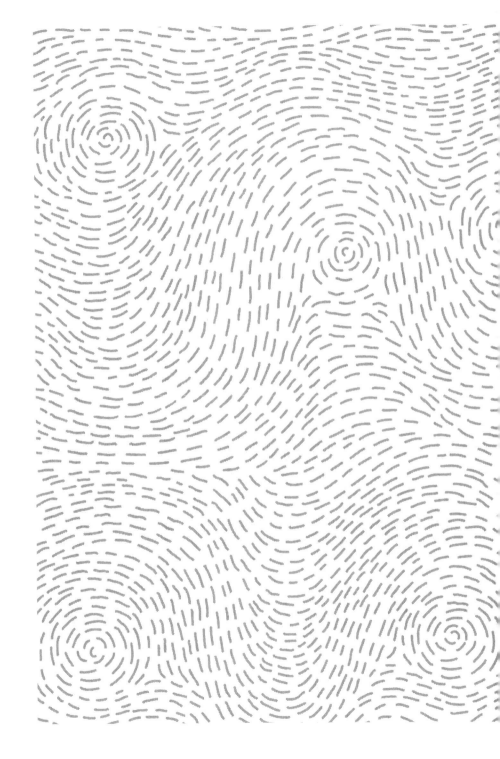

CHAPTER ELEVEN

Smoothies for Healthy Skin and Hair

While cosmetics can improve your looks temporarily, the secret to healthy skin and strong, shiny hair isn't in your makeup case. Glowing good looks are linked directly to your diet. Everything you consume becomes part of you at a cellular level. It affects the whole body, including the parts we can see: the hair, skin, and nails.

The more healthy food you consume, the healthier you will be, and that good health will show in your looks. The reverse is true, too. The less attention you pay to what you eat, the more difficulty you may have maintaining your looks.

If you're not getting the vitamins and minerals you need, you are essentially starving your body at a cellular level—and you're starving your skin and hair, too. While it takes time for poor eating habits to affect the way your hair looks, it can take as little as a week of bad food choices to make your skin look sallow and tired. Even worse, if your diet is missing vital nutrients for a long period of time, skin problems such as acne and eczema can result and hair can begin to thin.

Fortunately, eating a balanced diet with an abundance of natural foods can rapidly reverse these problems. Enjoy a green smoothie every day for a week and you will begin to see positive changes in your appearance. The recipes in this chapter have been created specifically to promote great-looking skin and beautiful hair.

Bunches of Blueberries

YIELDS 2 CUPS

Blueberries are among the foods highest in antioxidants, which protect the skin from premature aging. In addition, these tiny nutritional powerhouses contain high levels of vitamin K, vitamin C, and the essential mineral manganese. They are also an outstanding source of fiber. Eating as little as half a cup of blueberries daily can make a positive difference in the way you look.

1 CUP PURE AÇAI BERRY JUICE

1 BANANA, PEELED AND CUT INTO 1-INCH CHUNKS

1 CUP BLUEBERRIES

1 CUP CHOPPED GREEN OR RED LEAF LETTUCE, LOOSELY PACKED

Blend all ingredients together, pour into a tall glass, and enjoy. If you don't like açai berry juice, you can replace it with pure pomegranate juice or blueberry juice.

Spinach Spinner

Spinach is so high in antioxidants, minerals, and vitamins, including vitamin A, vitamin C, vitamin K, and vitamin E, that it's among the best foods for keeping your body's largest organ—the skin—looking good and functioning properly. The folate it contains contributes to a clear complexion, and the vitamins and antioxidants help repair damage. Spinach also contains iron, magnesium, calcium, and omega-3 fatty acids, all of which contribute to healthy hair growth.

1 CUP GREEN TEA, CHILLED

1 BANANA, PEELED AND CUT INTO 1-INCH CHUNKS

1 CUP STRAWBERRIES, HULLED AND HALVED

1 ORANGE, PEELED AND SEEDED

2 CUPS BABY SPINACH, LOOSELY PACKED

Blend all ingredients together, pour into a glass, and enjoy the delightful flavors of strawberries and citrus. If you'd like to add even more sumptuous fruit flavor while increasing your vitamin C intake, replace the green tea with fresh citrus juice.

Of all the liquids you can blend into green smoothies, green tea is one of the healthiest. Green tea contains powerful antioxidants called catechins, which fight cellular damage. These compounds also aid in lowering cholesterol and reducing blood pressure. Green tea has been shown to increase metabolism and stabilize blood sugar, making it the perfect replacement for sugary drinks. In addition, it helps improve blood flow, which is great for your skin and the rest of your body's structures. When making green tea, add water that's between 160–170°F. Boiling water kills the catechins in the tea. And don't overdo it. Have no more than 2 cups of caffeinated green tea daily and 2 cups of decaffeinated green tea, for a total of 4 cups a day at most.

. . . .

Banana-Walnut Wonder

YIELDS 3 CUPS

Walnuts contain high levels of omega-3 fatty acids, plus they are rich in vitamin E and biotin, both of which help strengthen hair and shield it from damage. Walnuts also contain plenty of copper, an essential mineral that helps impart luster and rich color to hair. While the walnuts in this recipe contain plenty of protein, the almond milk and alfalfa sprouts provide an additional boost of this essential nutrient.

1 CUP ALMOND MILK

2 BANANAS, PEELED AND CUT INTO 1-INCH CHUNKS

¼ CUP SHELLED WALNUTS

½ TEASPOON CINNAMON

¼ TEASPOON PURE VANILLA EXTRACT

½ CUP ALFALFA SPROUTS

10 ICE CUBES

Blend all ingredients together, pour into a glass, and savor the fantastic flavors of banana, nuts, cinnamon, and vanilla. Add more almond milk if the mixture is too thick for your taste. If you are craving a sweet, hearty treat, this luscious green smoothie is an excellent substitute for unhealthy options.

Greek Glory

Greek yogurt contains plenty of hair-friendly vitamin D, protein, and vitamin B_5, also known as pantothenic acid, and which is a popular ingredient in hair care products. Blueberries and spinach provide even more benefits to the hair and skin, while bananas offer creamy sweetness that counteracts the yogurt's tang.

1 CUP WATER

½ CUP PLAIN GREEK YOGURT

1 BANANA, PEELED AND CUT INTO 1-INCH CHUNKS

1 CUP BLUEBERRIES

1 CUP BABY SPINACH, LOOSELY PACKED

Blend all ingredients together, then pour into a glass and enjoy. If you'd like to add even more tangy fruit flavor while increasing your antioxidant intake, replace the banana with a cup of hulled strawberries.

Kiwi Crush

Kiwifruit contains high levels of vitamin C, which is essential for promoting healthy scalp circulation and supporting the tiny blood vessels that nourish your hair follicles. Fresh, zesty citrus fruits increase the amount of vitamin C this delightfully refreshing smoothie contains, and spinach provides numerous benefits as well.

1 CUP WATER

3 KIWIS, PEELED AND HALVED

1 ORANGE, PEELED AND SEEDED

1 TANGELO, PEELED AND SEEDED

1 CUP BABY SPINACH, LOOSELY PACKED

Blend all ingredients together, then pour into a glass and enjoy. If the consistency is too thin for your liking, add six ice cubes to the blender along with the spinach.

Mushroom Magic

Fresh mushrooms have an incredibly mild flavor, and they contain several important vitamins and minerals that help build healthy skin and hair. Mushrooms are one of just a handful of natural sources of vitamin D, which is vital for keeping teeth, bones, and skin healthy. They also contain high levels of biotin, pantothenic acid, and riboflavin, all of which contribute to strong, shiny hair and glowing skin.

1 CUP WATER

½ CUP WHITE OR CREMINI MUSHROOMS, WELL CLEANED

¼ AVOCADO, PEELED AND SEEDED

1 BANANA, PEELED AND CUT INTO 1-INCH CHUNKS

½ CUP HONEYDEW MELON, PARED, SEEDED, AND CUT INTO CHUNKS

1 TABLESPOON LOCAL HONEY

1 CUP BABY SPINACH, LOOSELY PACKED

Blend all ingredients together, then pour into a glass and enjoy. If you'd like to increase your smoothie's fruit flavor while boosting your antioxidant intake, replace the water with fresh citrus juice or some citrus-flavored herbal tea.

Blackberry Buzz

Blackberries are not just tasty; they are among the most powerful antiwrinkle foods nature provides. With high levels of antioxidants to fight the free radicals that contribute to skin damage, plus anti-inflammatory bioflavonoids and flavonoids, these juicy morsels also contain vitamin E in abundance. Almond milk nourishes with protein, while honey adds just a little extra sweetness.

1 CUP ALMOND MILK

2 CUPS BLACKBERRIES

1 TABLESPOON LOCAL HONEY

1 CUP CHOPPED BUTTER LETTUCE, LOOSELY PACKED

6 ICE CUBES

Blend all ingredients together, pour into a glass, and enjoy. This recipe works equally well with fresh or frozen blackberries. You can also get some of the same skin-strengthening benefits by using blueberries or a frozen berry medley with no sugar added.

Plum Passion

YIELDS 3 CUPS

Plums have a pleasant, tart flavor and contain plenty of vitamin A, vitamin C, and antioxidants that benefit skin. These delicious fruits are typically available only for a short time each summer in most places. They taste best and are most nutritious when consumed within a few days of being picked.

1 CUP WATER

1 BANANA, PEELED AND CUT IN 1-INCH CHUNKS

4 PLUMS, SEEDED AND QUARTERED

½ CUP CHOPPED BABY BOK CHOY

6 ICE CUBES

Blend all ingredients together and pour into a glass. If plums are not available, replace them with dark berries or purple grapes, which contain many of the same skin-friendly nutrients.

* *

Often referred to as Chinese cabbage, bok choy has smooth, upright leaves with bulbous white bottoms. You could almost say that bok choy has negative calories, because it takes more energy to digest than the plant contains. Bok choy is an excellent source of vitamin A, vitamin C, vitamin K, and many B-complex vitamins. It is also high in important antioxidants, including compounds that have been linked to the prevention of colon, prostate, and breast cancer. With numerous minerals, it is also excellent for circulatory health, which aids in promoting a look of youthful vitality. Baby bok choy has a milder taste than full-grown bok choy, which is why it is used in many smoothie recipes. But if you enjoy the taste of mature bok choy on its own, you will probably like it in smoothies too. Like other members of the cabbage family, bok choy contains chemical compounds called goitrogens, which can cause thyroid gland swelling in some individuals with thyroid disease.

Flaxseed Fantasy

YIELDS 2 CUPS

Flaxseed is very high in essential fatty acids, which are responsible for building healthy cell membranes. Your body's cell membranes aid in propelling nutrients into cellular structures and facilitating the expulsion of the waste cells produce. They also help hold water in while keeping toxins out. The stronger your skin's cell membranes, the more water they can hold, resulting in plump, younger-looking skin.

1 CUP ALMOND MILK

1 BANANA, PEELED AND CUT INTO 1-INCH CHUNKS

1 CUP RASPBERRIES

1 TABLESPOON FLAXSEED, SOAKED IN WATER FOR 30 MINUTES

½ CUP ALFALFA SPROUTS

Blend all ingredients together, then pour into a glass and enjoy. If you don't like almond milk, you can use any other type of milk: Coconut, soy, oat, and dairy milk all work well in this recipe.

Brazilian Beauty

YIELDS 2 CUPS

Brazil nuts are very high in selenium, an essential mineral that plays a key role in skin health. In clinical trials, people who consumed foods rich in selenium were less likely to suffer the type of oxidative skin damage that occurs when skin is sunburned. The mangoes in this recipe add tart sweetness and plenty of skin-boosting vitamin A and vitamin C.

1 CUP WATER

1 BANANA, PEELED AND CUT INTO 1-INCH CHUNKS

1 MANGO, PEELED, SEEDED, AND CUT INTO CHUNKS

¼ CUP BRAZIL NUTS, ROUGHLY CHOPPED

1 CUP CHOPPED GREEN OR RED LEAF LETTUCE, LOOSELY PACKED

Blend all ingredients together, pour into a glass, and enjoy this sweet, creamy green smoothie. If you don't like mango, or if it is not readily available, try using another yellow or orange fruit, such as papaya, peach, or apricot, to make this recipe your own.

Green Tea Slushie

Green tea protects the skin's cell membranes and has polyphenols with anti-inflammatory properties. Studies have shown that when taken orally or applied to the skin, green tea can even reduce the risk of damage caused by ultraviolet light, thus reducing the risk of skin cancer. The fruits and vegetables this smoothie contains add important vitamins and minerals to your diet.

1 CUP GREEN TEA, CHILLED

1 MANGO, PEELED, SEEDED, AND CUT INTO CHUNKS

1 CUP PAPAYA, PEELED, SEEDED, AND CUT INTO CHUNKS

1 CUP CHOPPED ROMAINE LETTUCE, LOOSELY PACKED

8 ICE CUBES

Blend all ingredients together, pour into a glass, and enjoy. If you'd like to add even more beneficial green tea to this smoothie, make ice cubes with the tea and use them in place of ice made with plain water.

CHAPTER TWELVE

Green Energy

Many people mistakenly believe that only foods that are dense in calories provide abundant energy. But many calorie-laden foods actually make you feel sluggish and contribute to obesity and chronic illness. In addition, many of today's favorite processed foods fail to supply essential micronutrients, which the body requires for energy conversion.

In contrast, there are many natural foods that feed your body, your brain, and even your heart. For example, blueberries and other dark fruits, such as blackberries and purple grapes, help keep the brain properly oxygenated, which in turn helps promote feelings of alertness while ensuring the body's ability to carry out essential tasks with efficiency.

All nutrients are important, but some play particularly vital roles in ensuring the body is able to use calories efficiently and function properly. Foods such as spinach, broccoli, and walnuts make the grade. So do citrus fruits like oranges and grapefruit; coconut; and avocado. Even humble oats are among the best foods for lasting energy and good health. The recipes in this chapter are designed to fill you up and give you the energy you need to live an active, happy life.

Avocado Envy

YIELDS 2 CUPS

Avocados satiate hunger because they contain plenty of healthy monounsaturated fat. While it's important to watch fat calories, our bodies do need fat to access certain fat-soluble vitamins, including vitamin A, vitamin K, vitamin E, and vitamin D. Avocados are also high in potassium and B vitamins, so don't be afraid to enjoy a little avocado each day. As an added bonus, your ability to turn down unhealthy choices improves when you're not feeling hungry.

1 CUP FRESH ORANGE JUICE

1 BANANA, PEELED AND CUT INTO 1-INCH CHUNKS

¼ AVOCADO, PEELED AND SEEDED

1 CUP STRAWBERRIES, HULLED AND HALVED

1 CUP CHOPPED GREEN OR RED LEAF LETTUCE, LOOSELY PACKED

Blend all ingredients together, pour into a glass, and enjoy. This rich-tasting smoothie is ideal as a meal replacement shake, particularly if you add a scoop of your favorite protein powder to the blender along with the lettuce.

Many varieties of strawberries are grown throughout the world, and each has a slightly different flavor and nutritional profile. All strawberries, however, are very low in calories, and all are an excellent source of vitamin C and vitamin A. In addition, strawberries are high in antioxidants, B-complex vitamins, folic acid, riboflavin, and pantothenic acid, which aid the body in effectively metabolizing proteins, fats, and carbohydrates. Certain individuals are sensitive to strawberries; they can cause hives, eczema, itching, swelling of the mouth and tongue, and other symptoms. If you suspect you may be allergic to strawberries, it's best to avoid them.

Spinach Swirl

Spinach contains plenty of energy-boosting B vitamins, including folic acid, plus it is loaded with other vitamins and important trace minerals. It's also a good source of omega-3 fatty acids, and it contains the calcium and magnesium necessary to build strong bones capable of supporting strenuous activity.

1 CUP GREEN TEA, CHILLED

1 BANANA, PEELED AND CUT INTO 1-INCH CHUNKS

1 CUP FROZEN STRAWBERRIES

1 CUP FROZEN MANGO CHUNKS

1 CUP BABY SPINACH, LOOSELY PACKED

Blend all ingredients together, pour into a glass, and enjoy this refreshing energy booster. You can replace the strawberries and mango chunks with other fruit combinations if you like. Pineapple, papaya, and peaches are all fantastic fruits to try, either fresh or frozen.

Fig Frenzy

Dried figs are relatively high in calories, but they make an outstanding addition to green smoothies that are designed to deliver lasting energy. They contain more fiber than any other vegetable or fruit, they are packed with vitamin B_6, and they complement many flavor combinations.

1 CUP ALMOND MILK

1 BANANA, PEELED AND CUT INTO 1-INCH CHUNKS

2 CUPS RASPBERRIES

¼ CUP DRIED FIGS, ROUGHLY CHOPPED

¼ TEASPOON PURE VANILLA EXTRACT

1 CUP ALFALFA SPROUTS

Blend all ingredients together, then pour into a glass and enjoy. If you can get fresh figs and would like to use them in this smoothie, you'll find the taste is slightly lighter yet just as pleasing.

Broccoli Blast

Broccoli contains many important micronutrients, along with magnesium, iron, and calcium. It also offers vitamins A and C, which are powerful antioxidants. The fiber it contains helps you feel full longer while slowing the absorption of the fruit sugars in this recipe.

1 CUP CITRUS-FLAVORED HERBAL TEA, CHILLED

1 BANANA, PEELED AND CUT INTO 1-INCH CHUNKS

1 CUP BROCCOLI FLORETS

1 CUP PAPAYA, PEELED, SEEDED, AND CUT INTO CHUNKS

4 TANGERINES, PEELED AND SEEDED

Blend all ingredients together, then pour into a glass and enjoy. If herbal tea isn't readily available, try using fresh citrus juice instead. You can also increase appeal by freezing the banana and papaya, or adding up to eight ice cubes to the blender after incorporating the tangerine.

. . . .

Broccoli is an autumn vegetable that is now widely available year-round. Extremely low in calories but rich in fiber, vitamins, minerals, and antioxidants, with proven health benefits, it has been shown to aid in preventing bladder, colon, prostate, breast, and pancreatic cancers. Although broccoli florets are most commonly consumed, the stems and leaves are also highly nutritious. The leaves contain high levels of vitamin A and carotenoids, and though they have an intense flavor with a strong bitter note, they may be added to green smoothies if you wish. As with other members of the cruciferous plant family, broccoli contains compounds called goitrogens that can cause the thyroid gland to swell in people who suffer from thyroid dysfunction. If you have thyroid disease, it's best to leave broccoli off the menu.

Instant Energy

YIELDS 2 CUPS

Bananas contain a trio of natural sugars: fructose, sucrose, and glucose. They also contain plenty of fiber, so the sugars are absorbed at a slow, even rate. If you're looking for a great green smoothie to help you power your way through a challenging workout or a boring afternoon meeting, this is an excellent one to try.

1 CUP ALMOND MILK

1 BANANA, PEELED AND CUT INTO 1-INCH CHUNKS

2 PEACHES, PITTED AND QUARTERED

1 CUP CHOPPED ROMAINE LETTUCE, LOOSELY PACKED

Blend all ingredients together, pour into a glass, and enjoy. This recipe tastes wonderful as is, but you can add half a teaspoon of cinnamon to give it a warm, satisfying flavor that can tame cravings for sweets.

Grape Green Machine

YIELDS 2 CUPS

Grapes contain powerful antioxidants, including vitamin C, and their sugar provides quick energy. The avocado in this recipe adds just the right amount of healthy fat to keep you feeling full for a few hours, and the spinach offers vitamins, minerals, and even more of the fiber your body needs.

1 CUP WATER

1 BANANA, PEELED AND CUT INTO 1-INCH CHUNKS

¼ AVOCADO, PEELED AND SEEDED

1 CUP GREEN GRAPES

1 CUP BABY SPINACH, LOOSELY PACKED

Blend all ingredients together for a sweet, creamy treat, adding a little more water if it is too thick. Pour into a glass and enjoy. If you prefer smoothies with tart flavors, add a tablespoon of lemon or lime juice to the blender after incorporating the spinach.

Cucumber-Melon Cooler

YIELDS 4 CUPS

Though cucumbers and melons are relatively low in calories, they contain essential nutrients, including the vitamins and minerals your body needs for lasting energy. Grapes add calories for energy, while bok choy imparts a fiber boost.

2 CUPS WATER

2 CUPS HONEYDEW MELON, PARED, SEEDED, AND CUT INTO CHUNKS

3-INCH CUCUMBER SEGMENT, UNPEELED, WELL WASHED, AND SLICED

½ CUP GREEN GRAPES

1 CUP CHOPPED BABY BOK CHOY

8 ICE CUBES

Blend all ingredients together, pour into a glass, and savor. If you prefer icy smoothies, try freezing the grapes and honeydew melon chunks before making this recipe.

Chocolate Almond Crunch

YIELDS 2 CUPS

Nuts and nut milks, including the almonds and almond milk in this recipe, provide the fat, protein, and calories required for energy. While chocolate is often viewed as an enemy of healthy eating, natural cacao nibs actually contain powerful antioxidants and an abundance of fiber, along with important minerals and micronutrients.

1½ CUPS ALMOND MILK

1 BANANA, PEELED AND CUT INTO 1-INCH CHUNKS

¼ CUP CACAO NIBS

1 TABLESPOON LOCAL HONEY

¼ CUP RAW OR BLANCHED ALMONDS

1 CUP ALFALFA SPROUTS

Blend all ingredients together, making sure you take extra care to incorporate the nuts and cacao nibs, then pour into a glass and enjoy. If cacao nibs are not available in your area, you can use 3 tablespoons of natural cocoa powder to replace them. To make the powder easier to incorporate, roll the banana chunks in it before adding them to the blender.

Chocolate comes from the bean of a plant. While processed chocolate candy, with added fat and sugar, is a treat to be savored occasionally, natural cacao nibs and cocoa powder contain high levels of dietary fiber, along with an antioxidant called flavanol that dilates blood vessels and increases blood flow to the brain, enhancing alertness. In addition, it provides some of the same benefits as hypertension drugs called ACE inhibitors, which decrease the potential for stroke. While natural cacao is high in calories and contains natural fat, it is an excellent ingredient to include in green smoothies a few times each week. Benefits are linked to regular consumption, so drink your chocolate.

Kiwi-Broccoli
Green Machine

YIELDS 4 CUPS

Kiwi, broccoli, kale, and apples contain an abundance of fiber that helps prevent sugar from being absorbed too rapidly. These fruits and vegetables also provide plenty of antioxidants, including vitamins A and C, which help protect the body's cells from oxidative damage, while ensuring nutrients are readily absorbed for lasting energy.

1½ CUPS WATER

1 BANANA, PEELED AND CUT INTO 1-INCH CHUNKS

1 APPLE, CORED AND CUT INTO CHUNKS

1 KIWI, PEELED AND HALVED

1 CUP BROCCOLI FLORETS

½ CUP FROZEN MANGO CHUNKS

1 CUP CHOPPED KALE, LOOSELY PACKED

8 ICE CUBES

Blend all ingredients together, pour into a glass, and enjoy the tart, delicious taste of this superb smoothie. Add more water if needed, as this recipe makes a thick, creamy frozen treat. Increase its protein content by incorporating almond milk, oat milk, or soy milk in place of the water.

Coconut-Cashew Champion

Coconut water contains high levels of electrolytes, making it the perfect choice for revitalizing the body after intense exercise or on a particularly hot day. When combined with fruit, nuts, and greens, it delivers optimal nutrition while providing energy that lasts.

1 CUP COCONUT WATER

1 BANANA, PEELED AND CUT INTO 1-INCH CHUNKS

1 CUP PINEAPPLE, CUT INTO CHUNKS

¼ CUP RAW OR BLANCHED CASHEWS

½ CUP ALFALFA SPROUTS

Blend all ingredients together, taking extra care to ensure the cashews are completely incorporated. Pour into a glass and enjoy. Transform this creamy smoothie into a frozen tropical treat by freezing the banana and pineapple chunks ahead of time.

Spiced Pumpkin Punch

YIELDS 4 CUPS

Pumpkin seeds have a lightly sweet taste that's irresistible, plus they contain high amounts of important trace minerals, including manganese, phosphorus, and magnesium, vital to healthy brain function. Pumpkin seeds also contain plenty of iron, protein, and fiber that can make any smoothie more nutritious.

1½ CUPS ALMOND MILK

1 BANANA, PEELED AND CUT INTO 1-INCH CHUNKS

1 TABLESPOON TOASTED PUMPKIN SEEDS

1 APPLE, CORED AND CUT INTO CHUNKS

¼ TEASPOON PURE VANILLA EXTRACT

½ TEASPOON CINNAMON

½ CUP CHOPPED BUTTER LETTUCE, LOOSELY PACKED

Blend all ingredients together, pour into a glass, and enjoy. If you'd like to add even more spicy flavor to this delicious smoothie, add half a teaspoon of ginger and a pinch of nutmeg.

CHAPTER THIRTEEN

Low-Fat Smoothies

While it is vital to eat enough healthy fat each day, it is also important to watch your overall fat intake. Fat contains 9 calories per gram, while carbohydrates and protein each contain 4 calories per gram. But simply eliminating fat—or adding it—will not leave you with a balanced diet. Whether you are trying to lose weight or maintain your weight, or even if you are attempting to gain weight in a healthy manner, it's vital to follow an eating plan that includes an abundance of vitamins and minerals, along with enough calories to prevent your body from dropping into starvation mode.

When the body takes in more fat than needed—even healthy monounsaturated fat from avocados and nuts—there is increased risk of developing a whole host of chronic health conditions. These include obesity, diabetes, high blood pressure, heart disease, and disorders that affect the kidneys and liver. The simple reason is that when excess calories are taken in the form of fat, the fat is readily transformed into body fat that is deposited deep in the abdomen, inside the arteries, and beneath the skin.

The recipes in this chapter are perfect for enjoying anytime, whether you have overdone it at a recent meal or are hoping to counteract poor food choices made over a long period of time. Don't worry. These delightful options for lower-fat smoothies are just as tasty as the more robust recipes other chapters contain.

Blackberry Peach Punch

YIELDS 4 CUPS

Bananas, blackberries, peaches, strawberries, and spinach contain no fat, yet they offer an abundance of important nutrients, including vitamins, minerals, and antioxidants. If you are rotating greens and it's not time to put spinach on the menu, feel free to replace it with any other greens you wish.

1 CUP WATER

1 BANANA, PEELED AND CUT INTO 1-INCH CHUNKS

1 CUP STRAWBERRIES, HULLED AND HALVED

1 CUP BLACKBERRIES

1 PEACH, PITTED AND QUARTERED

1 CUP BABY SPINACH, LOOSELY PACKED

Blend all ingredients together, then pour into a tall glass and enjoy. To add protein to this smoothie, replace half a cup of water with any nonfat milk, or add half a cup of nonfat plain yogurt or dairy-free yogurt.

• •

Like other dark berries, blackberries contain high levels of vitamins, minerals, and antioxidants, as well as plenty of dietary fiber. They also contain high levels of phytochemicals, including tannin, quercetin, and catechins, which have the potential to keep serious illness, including heart disease, cancer, and neurological disease, at bay. These compounds are also powerful antiaging and anti-inflammatory agents. Blackberries are rich in minerals, including copper, manganese, and potassium, and they are a good source of B vitamins. Some individuals are sensitive to the salicylic acid blackberries contain. It can lead to itching and swelling around the mouth, hives, eczema, and other unpleasant side effects. If you are allergic salicylic acid (the active ingredient in aspirin), blackberries are best avoided.

Cherry-Vanilla Cooler

YIELDS 4 CUPS

Although cherries and vanilla make their way into some of the world's most decadent desserts, it is possible to enjoy them without burdening your body with excess fat. Cherries are high in antioxidants, vitamins, and minerals, and nonfat yogurt contains plenty of protein for lasting satisfaction.

1 CUP WATER

1 CUP PLAIN NONFAT YOGURT

2 CUPS FROZEN CHERRIES

¼ TEASPOON PURE VANILLA EXTRACT

1 CUP ALFALFA SPROUTS

Blend all ingredients together, adding a bit more water if the mixture is too thick. Pour into a tall glass and enjoy. When shopping for frozen cherries, be sure to choose those that come already pitted and contain no added sugar.

Apple Chai Chiller

YIELDS 3 CUPS

Chai tea is a healthy alternative to coffee, containing an average of one-third less caffeine per cup. With its delicious spices and intrinsic sweetness, this comforting tea is perfect for low-fat smoothies. The nonfat yogurt this recipe contains provides an abundance of protein, while the apple provides a hint of sweet, fruity flavor that's sure to please your palate.

1 CUP UNSWEETENED CHAI TEA, CHILLED

1 CUP PLAIN NONFAT YOGURT

1 APPLE, CORED AND CUT INTO CHUNKS

¼ TEASPOON PURE VANILLA EXTRACT

½ CUP CHOPPED BUTTER LETTUCE, LOOSELY PACKED

Blend all ingredients together, pour into a glass, and enjoy. If you find that your smoothie is not sweet enough for your taste, add up to 1 tablespoon of local honey or a few drops of natural stevia extract.

Ginger Peach Greenie

Ginger has a warm, appealing taste that adds flavor to sweet and savory foods alike. Peaches and apricots impart delicious taste, and greens contain plenty of fiber to help you feel full. This fat-free smoothie is also very low in calories, so you can enjoy it any time you have a desire for something sweet and spicy.

1½ CUPS GINGER TEA, CHILLED

½ BANANA, PEELED AND CUT INTO 1-INCH CHUNKS

1 PEACH, PITTED AND QUARTERED

2 APRICOTS, PITTED AND HALVED

¼ TEASPOON GINGER

¼ TEASPOON PURE VANILLA EXTRACT

1 CUP CHOPPED BABY BOK CHOY

1 CUP BABY SPINACH, LOOSELY PACKED

Blend all ingredients together, pour into a glass, and sip to your heart's content. If you find the ginger flavor is too strong, either replace the herbal tea with water or omit the added ginger.

Strawberry Rhubarb Pie

YIELDS 3 CUPS

Strawberries and ripe rhubarb offer tangy, satisfying sweetness that can put a halt to even the most vicious cravings. A hint of real vanilla tempers the sharp flavors, while skim milk and Greek yogurt provide protein for lasting satisfaction.

1½ CUPS SKIM MILK

½ CUP PLAIN NONFAT GREEK YOGURT

1 CUP STRAWBERRIES, HULLED AND HALVED

3-INCH RHUBARB SEGMENT, CHOPPED

¼ TEASPOON PURE VANILLA EXTRACT

1 TABLESPOON LOCAL HONEY

1 CUP CHOPPED BUTTER LETTUCE, LOOSELY PACKED

Blend all ingredients together, pour into a glass, and enjoy. If you don't eat dairy products, you can replace the yogurt with the same amount of dairy-free yogurt. If you are watching your sugar intake and prefer not to eat honey, use a few drops of natural stevia extract in its place.

While rhubarb is often considered to be a fruit, and makes its way into desserts such as pies and cobblers, it is actually a herbaceous vegetable with strong stalks that bear a slight resemblance to celery. Though low in calories, rhubarb is an excellent source of dietary fiber, antioxidants, minerals, and vitamins. With lutein for eye health and vitamin K for strong bones, it is a valuable addition to smoothies. Only rhubarb stalks should be consumed; the plant's wide green leaves contain unsafe levels of oxalic acid, which can sometimes contribute to kidney failure and has been linked to death in the most severe cases.

Chocolate-Covered Banana

While this smoothie contains more calories than some others in this chapter, it contains only 2 grams of fat—1 for each tablespoon of cocoa powder. Though very simple, this recipe is wonderfully creamy and delicious.

1½ CUPS SKIM MILK

1 BANANA, PEELED AND CUT INTO 1-INCH CHUNKS

2 TABLESPOONS COCOA POWDER

1 CUP BABY SPINACH, LOOSELY PACKED

8 ICE CUBES

Blend all ingredients together, adding a little more milk if the blender blades begin to stick. Spoon or pour into a glass and enjoy. To more easily incorporate the cocoa powder, roll the banana chunks in it before adding them to the blender.

Strawberry Sunrise

Strawberries are sweet and delicious, and they contain just 52 calories per cup. All the ingredients in this smoothie contain no fat. If you're looking for a healthy green smoothie to share with a friend, this is a fantastic one to start with.

1 CUP WATER

1 CUP STRAWBERRIES, HULLED AND HALVED

1 CUP PINEAPPLE, CUT INTO CHUNKS

1 CUP PAPAYA, PEELED, SEEDED, AND CUT INTO CHUNKS

1 ORANGE, PEELED AND SEEDED

½ CUP ALFALFA SPROUTS

Blend all ingredients together, adding a little more water if the mixture is too thick. Spoon or pour into a glass and enjoy. You can easily transform this colorful smoothie into a delightful frozen treat by freezing the strawberries, pineapple, and papaya beforehand.

Apple Fennel Frappé

YIELDS 2 CUPS

Often-overlooked fennel is a marvelous green plant that has a delicious licorice flavor. The abundant greens are feathery and work well in salads. The bulb is high in fiber and low in calories. It also contains folic acid, vitamin C, and an abundance of potassium. When blended with apple and pear, fennel creates an irresistible smoothie that will satisfy your craving for sweets.

1 CUP WATER

1 APPLE, CORED AND CUT INTO CHUNKS

1 PEAR, CORED AND CUT INTO CHUNKS

½ CUP FENNEL BULB, CHOPPED

6 ICE CUBES

Blend all ingredients together, then pour into a glass and enjoy the cool, unexpected flavor this refreshing smoothie has to offer. If you'd like to add even more antioxidants, use chilled green tea in place of the water.

Cranberry Delight

Pure cranberry juice is very high in vitamin C and other important nutrients, and it is excellent for bladder and urinary tract health. Here, the tart taste of cranberry is tempered by the smooth sweetness cantaloupe and honey provide, while the alfalfa sprouts add protein for lasting satisfaction.

1 CUP PURE CRANBERRY JUICE

2 CUPS CANTALOUPE, PARED, SEEDED, AND CUT INTO CHUNKS

1 TABLESPOON LOCAL HONEY

½ CUP ALFALFA SPROUTS

6 ICE CUBES

Blend all ingredients together. If you'd like to add even more fruit flavor while increasing vitamin C, replace the water with fresh citrus juice.

Summer Splendor

Make the most of fresh summer fruits while keeping fat and calories low. This nutritious smoothie offers plenty of vitamins, minerals, and fiber, along with an abundance of folate, thanks to the baby spinach. The green tea provides an antioxidant boost your body will appreciate.

1 CUP GREEN TEA, CHILLED
2 NECTARINES, PITTED AND CUT INTO CHUNKS
1 CUP CHERRIES
1 CUP BABY SPINACH, LOOSELY PACKED

Blend all ingredients together, pour into a glass, and enjoy. If you can get fresh cherries, be sure to remove the pits and stems before adding them to your blender. If you find yourself shopping for frozen ones, make sure you choose the kind with no pits and no added sugar.

Raspberry Zinger

YIELDS 4 CUPS

Fresh raspberries are an excellent source of fat-free nutrition, offering an abundance of minerals, vitamins, and micronutrients. Low in calories, high in fiber, and wonderfully delicious, they pair perfectly with sweet peaches and mild-tasting Bibb lettuce.

1½ CUPS WATER

2 CUPS RASPBERRIES

1 PEACH, PITTED AND QUARTERED

1 CUP CHOPPED BIBB LETTUCE, LOOSELY PACKED

Blend all ingredients together, pour into a glass, and savor the succulent flavors of fresh, ripe fruit. If fresh raspberries and peaches are not available, simply use frozen ones. When shopping, be sure to select a brand that contains no added sugar.

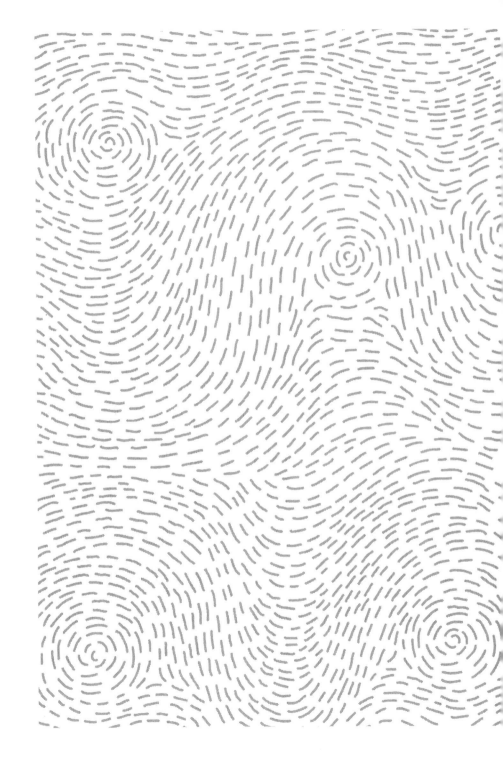

CHAPTER FOURTEEN

Green Smoothies Kids Will Love

If you are struggling to get the children in your life to eat enough vegetables and fruit, you'll find green smoothies are an excellent way to disguise ingredients they might not normally be willing to eat. By combining familiar flavors kids enjoy with healthy greens, then presenting these delicious concoctions in a fun way, you can easily convince even the most dedicated junk-food eater to give green smoothies a try.

Before attempting to convince your kids to drink green smoothies, be sure they see you and other adults enjoying them. Once you're ready to begin making the kids their own smoothies, allow them to get involved with preparing the fruits and vegetables that will go into the blender. If kids are old enough, allow them to push the buttons, too. This will give them a sense of ownership and increase their enthusiasm for trying these delicious treats.

Once your children have become accustomed to the green smoothies in this chapter, consider introducing them to the "grown-up" blends in other chapters. The more flavors they try, the more they are likely to be willing to eat new fruits and vegetables. By making green smoothies fun and exciting, you will open your children up to a whole new world of good health.

Green Banana

YIELDS 2 CUPS

*Most kids love bananas, even if they turn away from other fruits and vege-
tables. This delicious banana smoothie is an appealing light-green color.
Once your child becomes accustomed to drinking green smoothies, consider
gradually adding more greens.*

1 CUP WHOLE MILK

1 BANANA, PEELED AND CUT INTO 1-INCH CHUNKS

1 TEASPOON LOCAL HONEY

¼ CUP ALFALFA SPROUTS

Blend all ingredients together, incorporating additional milk if the mixture
is too thick. Pour into a cup and watch your little one enjoy. If milk isn't
part of your child's eating plan, use another liquid in its place. Nut milk, oat
milk, and orange juice are all good substitutes.

Monster Mash

YIELDS 3 CUPS

Once your child is ready to try a deep-green smoothie, it's time for this delicious concoction. Not only does it contain lots of tasty green fruit, but it hides a kid-size helping of broccoli along with a serving of raw spinach.

1 CUP WATER

2 KIWIS, PEELED AND HALVED

1 CUP GREEN GRAPES

1 GREEN APPLE, CORED AND CUT INTO 1-INCH CHUNKS

¼ CUP BROCCOLI FLORETS

½ CUP BABY SPINACH, LOOSELY PACKED

Blend all ingredients together, then serve in your child's favorite cup. If you'd like to add even more zippy fruit flavor while increasing your child's vitamin C intake, replace the water with fresh citrus juice.

Peanut Butter Sandwich

YIELDS 2 CUPS

Most kids love peanut butter and will enjoy the pleasant, nutty taste this smoothie offers. The wheat germ this recipe contains provides a healthy omega-3 boost, and the sprouts add even more protein while ensuring the blend isn't too green for smoothie novices.

1 CUP ALMOND MILK

1 BANANA, PEELED AND CUT INTO 1-INCH CHUNKS

1 PEAR, CORED AND CUT INTO CHUNKS

2 TABLESPOONS PEANUT BUTTER

1 TABLESPOON WHEAT GERM

¼ CUP ALFALFA SPROUTS

Blend all ingredients together, pour into a cup, and serve. If your kids like bright-green smoothies, feel free to replace the sprouts with other greens.

Disappearing Greens

YIELDS 3 CUPS

Bright red fruits do a great job of disguising healthy greens. Your kids will enjoy watching the greens disappear into the blender; the frozen berries and dark purple grape juice in this recipe do an excellent job of hiding them. Even the pickiest eater is sure to be impressed.

1 CUP PURE GRAPE JUICE

1 CUP FROZEN STRAWBERRIES

1 CUP FROZEN BLUEBERRIES

½ CUP CHOPPED ROMAINE LETTUCE, LOOSELY PACKED

Blend all ingredients together, then pour into a fun cup and present to your child. You can easily transform this recipe into a purple protein shake by adding a scoop of protein powder along with the lettuce.

Romaine lettuce contains few calories and has such a mild taste that it does not alter the flavor of smoothies at all. Even so, it contains plenty of fiber, vitamins, minerals, and antioxidants, making it a valuable addition to smoothies of all kinds, especially those created with picky kids in mind.

Orange Flip

Most picky eaters don't mind oranges and other citrus fruits, and nearly everyone likes bananas. The carrot adds vitamins, minerals, and an even brighter orange color kids will love, and the alfalfa sprouts disappear completely while providing a little satisfying protein that will keep hunger at bay until mealtime.

1 CUP FRESH ORANGE JUICE

1 BANANA, PEELED AND CUT INTO 1-INCH CHUNKS

2-INCH CARROT SEGMENT, PEELED AND THINLY SLICED

1 ORANGE, PEELED AND SEEDED

½ CUP ALFALFA SPROUTS

Blend all ingredients together, pour into a cup, and watch your child enjoy fresh fruits and vegetables. If you'd like to decrease the amount of sugar in the recipe, replace the orange juice with water. Once your child becomes accustomed to green smoothies, try adding spinach, kale, and other bright greens along with the alfalfa sprouts.

Pineapple Punch

Pineapple contains lots of fiber, plenty of antioxidants, and an abundance of vitamins and minerals. It tastes fantastic, too. The bananas provide a healthy dose of potassium, while the kale offers calcium, copper, iron, and lutein, which is essential for eye health.

1 CUP WATER

1 BANANA, PEELED AND CUT INTO 1-INCH CHUNKS

2 CUPS PINEAPPLE, CUT INTO CHUNKS

1 CUP CHOPPED KALE, LOOSELY PACKED

Blend all ingredients together, pour into a cup, and watch your child enjoying fresh greens. If your children are still learning to like green smoothies, use lighter greens: half a cucumber, half a cup of alfalfa sprouts, or half a cup of baby bok choy or Napa cabbage will provide a less vibrant look that won't intimidate timid eaters.

Tutti-Frutti

Thanks to tofu, this delicious green smoothie is high in protein, making it perfect for a quick meal on the go—minus anything even slightly resembling nuggets. Berries, banana, pineapple, and cucumber provide a healthy helping of fiber while ensuring your child gets the vitamins and minerals his or her growing body needs.

1 CUP WATER

½ CUP TOFU, DRAINED AND CUT INTO CUBES

1 BANANA, PEELED AND CUT INTO 1-INCH CHUNKS

1 CUP STRAWBERRIES, HULLED AND HALVED

1 CUP BLACKBERRIES

1 CUP PINEAPPLE, CUT INTO CHUNKS

3-INCH CUCUMBER SEGMENT, UNPEELED, WELL WASHED, AND SLICED

Blend all ingredients together, pour into a travel cup, and give your child a fantastic treat that's wonderfully healthy. If you'd like to add even more protein, replace the water with milk—dairy, oat, soy, or nut.

Green Lemonade

YIELDS 3 CUPS

Almost everyone enjoys fresh lemonade. This recipe contains an abundance of vitamins and minerals, no added sugar or artificial flavors, and a healthy helping of vibrant greens.

1 CUP WATER

3 ORANGES, PEELED AND SEEDED

JUICE FROM ½ LEMON

1 CUP CHOPPED RED OR GREEN LEAF LETTUCE, LOOSELY PACKED

Blend all ingredients together, pour into a cup, and serve. If you'd like to add even more fruit flavor while increasing the vitamin C, replace the water with fresh citrus juice.

Many people are surprised to discover that leaf lettuce is part of the daisy family. This delicious, light-flavored green has very few calories, but it contains high levels of nutrients, including vitamin A, vitamin C, and folate. In addition, it offers a wide array of minerals, including manganese, copper, and potassium, plus it is an excellent source of the B-complex vitamins that kids need for healthy development.

Brownie Blast

This decadent green smoothie is kid friendly, but it's also perfect for putting grown-up chocolate cravings to rest. The cocoa powder it contains is full of antioxidants and healthy fiber, while the bananas provide potassium, folate, vitamin B$_6$, and many other essential nutrients. Oats add a slightly nutty taste while giving the smoothie more body.

1 CUP ALMOND MILK

2 BANANAS, PEELED AND CUT INTO 1-INCH CHUNKS

¼ CUP COCOA POWDER

¼ CUP OATS

¼ TEASPOON PURE VANILLA EXTRACT

½ CUP BABY SPINACH, LOOSELY PACKED

8 ICE CUBES

Blend all ingredients together, adding more oat milk if the mixture is too thick. Pour into a cup and serve. Roll the banana pieces in cocoa powder to make incorporating the powder easier, and add a few drops of natural stevia extract if the smoothie isn't sweet enough.

Sugar Cookie

YIELDS 2 CUPS

It's almost impossible to resist a fantastic sugar cookie. This recipe will have your kids hooked on green smoothies in no time, and it's one you might find yourself enjoying, too. Almond milk provides protein, while bananas add just the right amount of sweetness. A touch of vanilla extract provides the perfect finishing touch.

1 CUP ALMOND MILK

2 BANANAS, PEELED AND CUT INTO 1-INCH CHUNKS

½ TEASPOON PURE VANILLA EXTRACT

½ CUP ALFALFA SPROUTS

Blend all ingredients together, pour into a glass, and serve. Add warm spices such as cinnamon and nutmeg to transform this healthy sugar cookie into an equally delicious snickerdoodle.

Chocolate-Covered Cherry

YIELDS 3 CUPS

Cherries and chocolate come together to create a timeless favorite everyone loves. The dark colors of the cherries and chocolate in this smoothie hide greens well, ensuring that even the most dedicated picky eater will enjoy this healthy treat without complaint.

1 CUP WATER

2 CUPS FROZEN CHERRIES

2 TABLESPOONS COCOA POWDER

½ CUP CHOPPED BABY BOK CHOY

Blend all ingredients together, adding more liquid if the mixture is too thick. Pour into a glass and serve. Roll the cherries in the cocoa powder before blending so the cocoa powder is easy to incorporate.

Know Your Produce

THE TOXIC TWENTY: WHAT TO BUY ORGANIC

Organic foods are almost always preferable to their conventionally grown counterparts, since no chemical fertilizers or pesticides are used to grow them. Sadly, it isn't always possible to find organic options. There are many conventionally produced foods that contain only low levels of these toxins, but there are several that contain levels so high that they're not really safe to eat unless they are organic.

The following toxic twenty foods should be consumed only if they are organic. If an ingredient isn't available organic, it's best to substitute another to keep yourself and your family safe.

Apples

Conventional growers use more than forty different pesticides on their apples, as insects and fungus threaten crops. Pesticide residue is found not just on fresh apples, but in apple products such as applesauce and apple juice. If you buy these items, choose organic.

Bell Peppers

Bell peppers are treated with almost fifty different pesticides intended to keep insects and fungus away. These thin-skinned vegetables are difficult to clean completely, so be sure to use only organic ones.

Blueberries

Blueberries might be powerfully nutritious, but conventionally grown varieties can't be trusted. Choose organic blueberries, even if that means you have to buy frozen ones. As a bonus, frozen varieties are easier to store and add cool goodness to smoothies.

Celery

Celery is heavily treated with pesticide, and that pesticide drips down into the plant's ribs. Tests conducted by the U.S. Depatrment of Agriculture (USDA) has found more than sixty different pesticides tainting celery.

Cherry Tomatoes

Bugs love to eat cherry tomatoes, and the fruit is also woefully susceptible to fungal attack. Cherry tomatoes are treated with a toxic cocktail of pesticides, making them one of the dirtiest plant foods on the market. Look for organic ones, and try growing your own during the summer.

Coffee

Coffee, including green coffee extract, sometimes makes its way into green smoothies, and many of us enjoy our morning cup of joe. To stay on the safe side, choose fair trade–certified and Rainforest Alliance–labeled organic coffee; it is grown without pesticides.

Collard Greens

Just like kale and spinach, healthy collard greens are often treated with a mind-boggling array of pesticides. The USDA has revealed that there are as many as forty-five different chemicals commonly used on collards. Organic collard greens can be found in many places. If you can't find them, try cabbage or Brussels sprouts instead.

Cucumbers

Cucumbers are among the dirtiest types of produce on the market, unless they're organic. More than thirty-five different pesticides are used to treat these green beauties. If you can't find organic ones, peeling the skin off will greatly reduce your chances of exposure, but it will also eliminate many of the plant's nutrients.

Grapes

Grapes are a favorite with people everywhere, but since they are susceptible to fungus and insect attack, farmers often raise them conventionally, using as many as thirty different pesticides in the process. Grapes should always be purchased organic; there's just no way to eliminate all the residue.

Hot Peppers

Hot peppers such as jalapeños are often coated in a toxic sheen of pesticide. Buy them organic, or don't buy them at all.

Kale

Yet another of the best leafy green vegetables for smoothies, kale is quite hardy, but conventional farmers treat it with pesticides anyway. Luckily, this popular plant is very easy to find in farmers markets and at grocery stores, proudly bearing an organic label.

Lettuce

Like other leafy green vegetables, lettuce is a favorite with bugs of all kinds, so conventional farmers resort to spraying it with a toxic blend of more than fifty different pesticides. Organic lettuce is very easy to find at grocery stores and in farmers markets, and it's very easy to grow in a container or in a small garden.

Meat

No one puts meat in smoothies, but what you eat when you aren't drinking smoothies is just as important as what makes its way into your glass. Since beef and other meat animals are given a steady diet of pesticide-laden food, the pesticides bioaccumulate inside their body fat, eventually making their way into your food. If you eat pork, beef, chicken, turkey, or other meat, select only organic options.

Milk

Like meat, milk contains high levels of pesticides. In fact, tests have shown as many as twelve different ones contaminating conventionally produced milk. Choose organic milk or select a nut or soy milk instead.

Nectarines

Nectarines, particularly those imported from other countries, are laced with as many as thirty-three different pesticides. Choose organic ones or select a different fruit to use in your smoothies.

Peaches

Like nectarines, peaches are covered in a toxic film of pesticides. Testing has shown more than sixty types of pesticides on peaches. Thanks to their fuzzy skin, peaches are particularly difficult to clean. Buy them organic, or select a different type of fruit.

Potatoes

Luckily, most people don't include potatoes in smoothies, but because these mineral-rich vegetables are a favorite at dinnertime, they make the list. Testing has shown there are more than thirty-five different pesticides used on potatoes, with russets being among the filthiest. Sweet potatoes are a good substitute.

Spinach

Unfortunately, one of the most reliable green smoothie ingredients has a constant presence on the toxic list. Often treated with as many as fifty different pesticides, this leafy green is impossible to clean and should be eaten only if it is organic. Fortunately, organic spinach, including many pre-washed and prepackaged options, is readily available at an affordable price.

Strawberries

Strawberries grow close to the ground and are susceptible to attack by both insects and fungal diseases. Farmers use almost sixty different pesticides to keep their berries from being ruined, and it's nearly impossible to get them completely clean. Choose organic strawberries, even if that means you have to buy them frozen rather than fresh.

Zucchini

This popular summer squash has a thin skin and is a favorite with pests, so conventional farmers use an array of pesticides to keep bugs away. Organic zucchini is easy to find and is a plant anyone can grow with minimal effort.

A GUIDE TO SEASONAL SHOPPING

As the seasons change, so do the items available at local farmers markets. While much depends on the seasons where you live, there are many fruits and vegetables that are best and freshest at certain times of the year.

Spring

Artichokes	Carrots
Arugula	Cauliflower
Asparagus	Cherries
Beets	Cilantro
Blueberries	Collard greens

Fennel
Fiddlehead ferns
Garlic
Green onions
Kale
Kohlrabi
Leeks
Lettuce
Mint
Mushrooms
Onions

Parsley
Pea sprouts
Peas
Potatoes
Rhubarb
Snow peas
Strawberries
Swiss chard
Turnip greens
Turnips

Summer

Apricots
Avocados
Basil
Beet greens
Beets
Bell peppers
Blackberries
Blueberries
Broccoli
Cantaloupe
Carrots
Cauliflower
Cherries
Cilantro
Collard greens
Corn
Fennel
Figs
Gooseberries

Green beans
Honeydew melon
Hot peppers
Kale
Lettuce
Nectarines
Peaches
Pears
Peas
Plums
Rhubarb
Snow peas
Summer squash
Swiss chard
Tomatoes
Watermelon
Zucchini

Autumn

Apples
Artichokes
Arugula
Beet greens
Beets
Belgian endive
Blackberries
Blueberries
Broccoli
Brussels sprouts
Butternut squash
Cauliflower
Celery
Celery root
Collard greens
Eggplant
Fennel
Figs
Garlic

Grapes
Kale
Kohlrabi
Lettuce
Parsnips
Pears
Persimmons
Potatoes
Pumpkins
Radicchio
Radishes
Rhubarb
Rutabagas
Spaghetti squash
Spinach
Sweet potatoes
Swiss chard
Tomatoes
Zucchini

Winter

Beet greens
Beets
Belgian endive
Broccoli
Brussels sprouts
Butternut squash
Cabbage
Carrots
Cauliflower
Celery

Celery root
Collard greens
Curly endive
Fennel
Garlic
Kale
Leeks
Onions
Parsnips
Persimmons

Potatoes

Pumpkins

Radicchio

Rutabagas

Spaghetti squash

Sweet potatoes

Turnip greens

Turnips

References

Dobbins, Lee Anne. *Healthy Smoothie Recipes: Healthy Herbal Smoothies That Are Nutritious, Delicious and Easy to Make.* Lee Anne Dobbins, 2012.

Pratt, Steven G., MD, and Kathy Matthews. *SuperFoods Rx: Fourteen Foods That Will Change Your Life.* New York: Harper, 2005.

Morris, Julie. *Superfood Kitchen: Cooking with Nature's Most Amazing Foods.* New York: Sterling Epicure, 2012.

Raiz, Gabrielle. *Green Smoothie Magic: 132+ Delicious Green Smoothie Recipes That Trim and Slim.* Gabrielle Raiz, 2012.

Rockridge University Press. *The Smoothie Recipe Book: 150 Smoothie Recipes, Including Smoothies for Weight Loss and Smoothies for Good Health.* Berkeley, CA: Rockridge Press, 2013.

Watson, Christine. *500 Smoothies and Juices: The Only Smoothies and Juices Compendium You'll Ever Need.* Portland, ME: Sellers Publishing, 2011.

Index

95216815R00113